AIDS-PROOFING YOUR KIDS

A STEP-BY-STEP GUIDE

LOREN E. ACKER, Ph.D.

BRAM C. GOLDWATER, Ph.D.

and

WILLIAM H. DYSON, M.D., Ph.D.

Beyond Words Publishing, Inc.

Published by
Beyond Words Publishing, Inc.
13950 NW Pumpkin Ridge Road
Hillsboro, Oregon 97123
Phone: (503) 647-5109
Toll-free: 1-800-284-9673

Editor: Michelle Roehm
Page Layout: The TypeSmith
Cover Design: Soga Design

Distributed to the book trade by Publishers Group West

The information contained in this book is intended to be educational and not
for diagnosis, prescription, or treatment of disease or of any health disorder
whatsoever. This information should not replace competent professional advice
and does not guarantee that a person will not contract HIV if they follow the
instructions in this book. The information provided in this book represents the
most current medical information available as of this date. The authors strongly
recommend that in addition to using the book the reader enrolls in a competent
sex- or AIDS-education class. The authors and Publisher are in no way liable
for any use or misuse of the the material. The groups listed in Chapter 10 are
for resource and information purposes only and these groups do not necessarily
endorse or recommend this book.

Library of Congress Cataloging-in-Publication Data

Acker, Loren E. (Loren Edward), 1936-
  AIDS-proofing your kids : a step-by-step guide / Loren E. Acker,
Bram C. Goldwater, and William H. Dyson.
      p.   cm.
  Includes bibliographical references.
  ISBN: 0-941831-72-8
  ISBN 13: 978-0-941831-72-7

  1. Sex instruction—United States. 2. Parent and teenager—United
States. 3. Safe sex in AIDS prevention—United States. 4. AIDS
(Disease)—United States—Prevention. I. Goldwater, Bram C. (Bram
Charles), 1942-   , II. Dyson, William H., 1943-   , III. Title.
HQ57.A28 1992
613.9'51—dc20   91-43490
                                                                   CIP

Dedicated to Today's Parents

It is our hope that more-effective parenting techniques may help you solve today's complex problems

Contents

About the Authors

Loren Edward Acker, Ph.D

Dr. Loren Acker was educated at the University of California and is currently a professor at the University of Victoria in British Columbia, Canada. Before teaching in Canada, he was an Overseas Research Fellow for the United States Public Health Service, developing behavioral teaching strategies for children and youths. Dr. Acker is presently teaching, doing research and professionally practicing in child psychology and behavior management. He is an active father of four, deeply involved with his kids' schooling and community activities.

Dr. Acker brings to this book two decades of professional experience in working with families, school classrooms, and community agencies. He is no stranger to the considerations and problems of parenting, education, and behavior development. His publications in scientific journals and books, his national television and radio appearances, and his invited lectures in North America and England have addressed the many problems of children growing up. Yet with all the scientific credentials and experience that Dr. Acker has acquired, he presents his knowledge in a down-to-earth, practical manner that has made him ever-popular with his students, audiences, and colleagues.

Dr. Acker dedicates his contributions in this book to his family, to their health and happiness, and to the well-being of all kids who must bravely face the coming decades.

Bram Charles Goldwater, Ph.D

Dr. Bram Goldwater was educated at McGill, Cornell, and Bowling Green universities and is currently a professor at the University of Victoria in British Columbia, Canada. He has been teaching the basic principles of learning for more than twenty years, bringing to it an avid interest in both the understanding of behavior and in the best ways to communicate that understanding to others. His other research and teaching interests include the physiological study of arousal and emotion, modification of bodily reactions, and the relationship between psychology and disease.

Dr. Goldwater's publications in leading scientific journals and his training of numerous doctoral students have given him a well-deserved reputation as a careful scholar and teacher in the analysis of behavior. Furthermore, his co-development, with Dr. Acker, of innovative instructional methods for the teaching of basic psychological principles to university students as well as to parents, teachers, and community personnel has given him the sensitivity and expertise that helps make this book readable and practical.

Dr. Goldwater dedicates his contributions in this book to his students who, over the years, have convinced him of the importance of the instructional principles on which this book is based.

William Hallman Dyson, M.D., Ph.D

Dr. William Dyson was educated at Moravian College, the University of Kansas, and McMaster University and is currently a professor and practicing physician at the University of Victoria in British Columbia, Canada. He has a strong background in basic science and was a well-published researcher in cell growth and differentiation prior to leaving the laboratory for clinical medicine. In the past decade he has fused his science background with clinical medicine while teaching for the School of Nursing at the university. The problem of AIDS has become a key topic in his courses over the years. Dr. Dyson has had to consider the basic science and develop the resulting clinical realities of this problem for purposes of effectively teaching his students. Dr. Dyson was appointed coordinator for policy on AIDS at the university, a policy that requires the institution of effective preventive programs for the university community.

Dr. Dyson practices medicine at the University Health Services and has more than a decade of experience in serving the medical needs of sexually active young people. Many of these young people are now parents themselves, and it is out of his compassion for all his past and future young patients that he dedicates his contributions in this book. It is his sincere hope that all will find a way to successfully face the formidable challenge of AIDS.

PART I

Introduction

1

Their Lives in Your Hands

The days when **Acquired Immune Deficiency Syndrome** (AIDS) was "someone else's" disease are over. It is not a virus that strikes only homosexuals and intravenous (IV) drug users anymore. Our children are now dying from it as well. We, as parents, cannot fool ourselves any longer — it's too dangerous for our kids.

By mid-1991, over 33,000 young Americans were dying of AIDS, and the majority of these became infected during their teen years.
— Centers for Disease Control, Atlanta

More than a quarter of our kids are sexually active by age 15.
— *U.S.A. Today,* October 7, 1991

20% of all people diagnosed with AIDS were likely infected during their teenage years.
— Oregon State Health and Statistics Group,
September 1991

7

You may figure that your kids are too young for sex to be a concern. Is a 10-year-old too young to worry about? Is a 20-year-old too old? No one can tell you, for sure, about your kids. You're in the best position to find out about your kids' knowledge about sex, their interest in sex, and the peer pressure they may be under to engage in sex. You'll have to devote time to them to do this:

- **To help you judge your kids' level of knowledge or experience,** listen to some of their unguarded or joking comments about sex and try to assess the depth of their understanding, their "worldliness." Look for misunderstandings, distortions, or just plain ignorance. How much of what they know can be attributed to direct experience as opposed to family or school educational sources?

- **To help you judge your kids' interest in sex,** watch a few of the teen- and preteen-oriented television shows that they're turning on, including family situation comedies. Are your kids showing a keen interest in the more sexually provocative shows and the more sexually provocative scenes? Do their comments, laughter, or embarrassments shed light on their interests and personal experiences?

- **To help you judge the peer pressure your kids are under,** look at the use of cosmetics and sexually provocative clothes at your local junior high school or middle school — and, perhaps, elementary school. To what extent are your kids conforming to these fashion codes? To what extent do they appear to resist or protest the popular fads through their words and actions?

You'll have to look and listen to appreciate that sex is the concern of preteens and teens alike, and their sexuality must be of importance to us if our concern about AIDS is real.

You may believe that your kids have learned enough about AIDS from the media and from sex-education classes in school to know how to take care of themselves or to be cautioned away from sex. If kids have learned a lot about AIDS, it sure hasn't made them cautious:

Risky sexual behavior is widespread among adolescents .... Several surveys have reported that approximately 60% of adolescents are engaging in risky behavior.
> — U.S. Office of Technology Assessment, 1988

Neither fear . . . nor knowledge about AIDS appeared to significantly influence the decision to abstain from coital activity.
> — Survey of more than 5,000 Canadian college students

And there's growing evidence that kids can't learn about AIDS effectively from others. It has to be up to you:

A growing number of family experts say that the best sex education is done at home.
> — Peter Jennings, ABC News

Watch out! No one else can likely get through to your kids. Think about this: If you have hesitations about dealing with your kids' risky sexual practices, you can imagine the cautious and less-than-candid approach that teachers may bring to your kids' sex-education classes. *You are your kids' best hope:*

Teens that participate in sex-education programs that involve their parents are half as likely to be sexually active.
— *U.S.A. Today,* October 7, 1991

If you are still relying on your kids to learn from others about sex and how to avoid getting AIDS, the facts are not encouraging. Consider the results of a recent survey of school-age kids:

FACT: Although approximately half the students worried about getting AIDS, only 15% of eleventh-grade students said this was keeping them from sexual intercourse.

FACT: Almost half the eleventh-grade students had had sexual intercourse at least once.

FACT: Forty percent were embarrassed to buy condoms.

FACT: Only 14% of first-year college and university students use condoms all the time.

You may be convinced that your kids are safe because their friends are "clean." No one in your kids' crowd could possibly be an AIDS carrier, right? How could you really know this? Even if this were true, it would take your kid or only one of your kids' friends to have a sexual contact outside that group — with an AIDS carrier infected through sexual abuse, drug experimentation, or contact with a prostitute — to put others in the group at risk.

That's why education and prevention are so important. But it is not enough that kids simply be exposed to information about their risks and options. Kids must be taught safe practices that they can actually adopt and follow. And this means that parents must teach them these skills thoroughly and effectively. As we said before, who else can do it? That's why we've written this book. We've brought to it an understanding of exactly how to promote optimal learning, an understanding that we've acquired over our many years in education, behavioral science, and medicine. Our goal is to provide you with step-by-step techniques to follow in teaching your kids to protect themselves from AIDS.

Some of you may question the message of this book, or parts of it, at least. Attitudes toward sexual behavior and to talking about or dealing directly with sexual behavior vary greatly. People disagree about what is desirable, what is acceptable, what is proper. But there can be no disagreement as to the need for effective ways to safeguard our kids as they enter their period of heightened sexual activity.

We are providing you with a wide range of options in this book, from coaching your kids in successfully *abstaining from sex* to getting down to the nitty-gritty of coaching them in the effective *use of condoms*. These AIDS-proofing "prescriptions" are unlikely to hurt you and your kids, yet they are very likely to help protect your kids from AIDS as well as from other sexually transmitted diseases and unplanned pregnancies. This book will foster a more open and improved communication between you and your kids about sex.

We hope you will give all our health "prescriptions" your serious consideration, because AIDS-proofing is possible and our kids need our help. Stick with us and we'll show you how!

2

Teaching Made Easy: Ensuring Your Success

This book is designed to help you prepare your kids to protect themselves from AIDS. We will spell out a variety of practical steps that you can take to help guard your kids from sexual transmission of the AIDS virus. We will help you AIDS-proof your kids, as painlessly as possible, showing you:

- **How to talk to your kids about AIDS** and to make certain that they fully appreciate the seriousness of the disease and understand which sexual behaviors put them at risk.

- **How to ensure that your kids will have a condom** when they need one, will apply it properly, and will be assertive so that neither shyness nor passion will deter them from using it.

- **How to coach your kids in saying "no"** — "no" to sex without a condom, or possibly "no" to any sex under any circumstances. We want you to help them learn how to be assertive enough to convince a stubborn partner, yet gentle enough to avoid provoking harsh reactions.

- **How to inform and counsel your kids** about ways of engaging in interpersonal sex without intercourse, so that they will know and accept safe and satisfying alternatives.

- **How to engage your kids in leisure activities** that avoid opportunities for interpersonal sex, because abstinence is also an important AIDS-proofing strategy.

We are going to give you concrete advice on what to do or say, including examples. Many of you will need this help, because not everyone is used to discussing sex freely with their kids — it's embarrassing or at least uncomfortable. Your kids probably won't jump at the chance to talk to you about these things, either. And like any safety practices, whether involving driving, using power tools, or handling dangerous household substances, safe sexual practices have to be learned well if they're to be effective. The skills you'll be teaching your kids will have to be learned soundly and thoroughly if they're to be counted on to protect their lives.

We are going to provide you with the most powerful and painless techniques available for teaching your kids. In each chapter, we'll outline a number of specific steps you can take (a) to reduce your own and your kids' discomfort at discussing sexual and (b) to maximize the effectiveness with which your kids learn protective sexual practices.

The instructional techniques below were developed by behavioral scientists and are easy to use in teaching all kinds of behavioral skills in homes and schools all around the world.

APPROVAL AND REWARD

Your kids probably won't be eager initially to have you teach them safe sexual practices. Their cooperation, no matter how minimal at first, must receive your generous praise, approval, and material rewards. Behavioral scientists know how important it is for kids to experience immediate, positive rewards for desirable behavior. We'll be stressing the importance of the principle of positive reinforcement throughout this book.

Be prepared to promise your kids rewards for their cooperation. The promised use of the car for that special date, or money put toward that long-wanted amplifier or pair of skis, or an evening of their choice of videos will help change their attitude and ensure their continued participation. Don't be offended by this — *it is not bribery!* Bribery is offering a reward to someone to do something that is not in their best interest, but rather in yours. You should feel confident and good about using approval and reward in AIDS-proofing your kids. After all, you work in a community that approves and rewards your efforts and labor. Your kids' efforts toward AIDS-proofing through safe sexual practices deserve at least this same support.

There is another important reason for our emphasis on approval and reward. Approval and reward make for positive feelings between you and your kids. Unfortunately, there are only two alternatives — both bad — to praising and rewarding kids for doing what's good for them. You can either ignore their habits, which, in the case of AIDS, could mean a death sentence, or punish them for their unsafe habits. But punishment, even when effective, can make for feelings of resentment and ill will between you and your kids. And let's face it, the last thing you want is to have your efforts at

AIDS-proofing, which may already be embarrassing, create negative feelings between you and your kids. So forget any use of threats, punishments, or other coercive ways that may have worked for you in the past. For AIDS-proofing, approval and reward are your best allies and should always be your course of action.

But your approval and rewards, by themselves, often will not be enough. Some things are just too embarrassing for your kids to talk about or too new and complicated for them to be able to do successfully. Applying a condom quickly and carefully to a sausage, as suggested in Chapter 4, may require more skill than your kids can presently manage, no matter how much praise and reward is offered. Similarly, if your kids lack the assertiveness needed to refuse to have sex, simply promising them greater rewards won't solve the problem. You'll need to use progressive coaching and realistic practice. When accompanied by lots of praise and reward, progressive coaching and realistic practice can promote effective and enjoyable learning.

PROGRESSIVE COACHING

Progressive coaching is a way to make even the most difficult task easier to do by reducing it to small, manageable steps. No matter how shy, inexperienced, or unskilled your kids may be, and no matter how uncomfortable you both may feel about discussing safer sex, progressive coaching can help.

The three keys to progressive coaching are *start small*, *progress gradually*, and *readjust expectations when necessary*. Here's how it works:

- **Start small.** In progressive coaching, you begin with a comfortable and simple task that your kids can do easily. This minimizes embarrassment, maximizes their first chance of success, and, most importantly, encourages them to continue trying.

- **Progress gradually.** Once the initial tasks are mastered, new, minimal challenges are added. Don't ask your kids to progress to the next, more difficult step until they've succeeded with what's at hand. Increase your expectations a little at a time so as to ensure continued success, continued praise, and continued reward.

- **Readjust expectations when necessary.** Learning new or embarrassing skills doesn't always progress smoothly. You have to watch for signs of difficulty and "back-off" as needed. For example, embarrassment or reluctance may increase with increasingly detailed conversations about sex. Fumbling or awkwardness may arise as a kid progresses from putting condoms onto a broom handle to putting them onto a sausage. In both cases, you must be patient and flexible enough to temporarily lower your expectations. You must fall back to a more comfortable conversation that contains less mention of sex, or to a simpler task, such as practicing putting the condom onto a cucumber before going on to the more difficult, flexible sausage. This will reinstate confidence, good feelings, and permit progress over the long term.

Here's another example of progressive coaching. If your kids were too embarrassed to buy condoms, in spite of your repeated requests:

- You'd have to **start small** with something they do feel able to do — such as just walking into the store and noting where the condoms are displayed.

- You'd **progress gradually** from there, perhaps next asking them to examine the brands in the display rack. Purchasing condoms would be a step they would take later on, another day perhaps, when they eventually feel comfortable enough to do so.

- But if their attempts at purchasing weren't successful, you'd be prepared to **lower your expectations**: "OK, then just go back and check out what brands are available at another pharmacy."

In a nutshell, progressive coaching ensures continued success by making sure you start at your kids' level of competence and that your expectations don't exceed their current ability. It's a way to maximize gain and minimize pain. And don't forget — the glue that holds progressive coaching together is the praise, approval, and encouragement that should accompany all attempts at learning new skills.

We'll provide you with progressive coaching techniques so you can help your kids acquire skills for practicing safer sex as well as for abstaining from sex. You'll also use these techniques to gradually overcome any embarrassment you and your kids may experience in the process.

THE RISKS OF NOT USING
PROGRESSIVE COACHING

We've all seen what can happen to our kids when teachers, coaches, and we, as parents, expect too much from them too quickly. Too often there is failure to provide praise for their first small, slow-to-develop accomplishments. We've seen how discouraged our kids can get when they don't keep up to the level expected of them. We've watched them get frustrated and disheartened when their performance on the playing field is devalued or ignored simply because it's not as good as it might be. We've seen kids give up on their schoolwork and after-school activities rather than continue to fall short of the expectations of others. With better instructional techniques, including lots of approval for all levels of achievement and progressive coaching to develop skills and confidence, you can be successful in teaching and motivating your child.

Our goal in the chapters that follow is to ensure your success when teaching your kids how to protect themselves from AIDS. Your kids can't afford to fail — the consequences may be far too serious.

REALISTIC PRACTICE

Learning new skills through progressive coaching isn't enough without your kids regularly practicing these skills under conditions as similar as possible to those where they'll ultimately apply them. The importance of practicing under realistic conditions is well-known. Top athletes, for example, practice under conditions similar to those under which they'll actually compete. Firefighters practice putting out fires under realistic, simulated conditions. And jet pilots are trained on sophisticated devices that simulate the conditions they'll encounter when actually flying.

The same principle applies to the skills you'll be teaching your kids. If, for example, your kids are to be able to refuse having sex without a condom or to refuse sex entirely, they'll have to get a great deal of practice in effective refusing. This practice should occur under conditions as similar as possible to those they'll encounter "out in the real world." Your kids won't be protected if they're perfectly knowledgeable about safe sexual practices when they talk to you, but fail to apply this knowledge in their sexual encounters. We'll show you how to develop and use role-playing for simulating the actual situations under which your kids will be protecting themselves from AIDS.

BE CONFIDENT — YOU'VE LIKELY DONE THIS BEFORE

Some of our recommended techniques may seem a little strange to you at first, but it's really nothing new. You've probably applied progressive coaching and realistic practice before, perhaps in teaching your older teenagers safety skills such as safe driving.

Safe driving, much like safer sex, involves doing the right thing at the right time in order to avoid harm. Most teenagers have the basic abilities needed to drive; it's getting them to apply specific skills properly and consistently that is the problem. This is the case for safe sexual behavior as well. To ensure that your kids learned to drive safely, you likely wanted them to get lots of practice with a number of proper driving behaviors and under varied traffic conditions. You wanted your kids to repeatedly and reliably demonstrate behaviors such as wearing a seat belt, slowing down before a stop sign or red light, signaling turns, and so on.

Of course, if your kids were a bit nervous about getting behind the wheel for the first time or if their coordination was a little weak, you may have used a bit of progressive coaching. You most likely started slow with some basic maneuvers under conditions completely removed from traffic. Later, when both you and your kids had more confidence in their ability, you gradually advanced to more demanding techniques and conditions.

You may also have used progressive coaching and realistic practice in teaching your kids how to say "no" to friends who urge them to drive less safely or who insist that they get into a car with a drinking driver.

We're asking you to apply these same techniques in teaching your kids the skills they'll need to protect themselves from AIDS. Each chapter provides specific procedures for you to follow, based on principles of progressive coaching and realistic practice. Your understanding of these techniques, along with the generous use of approval and reward, will help to ensure your success in AIDS-proofing your kids.

SOME WORDS OF CAUTION

- **Don't delay.** Encouraging trusting communication between you and your kids cannot begin too early. Even if you feel your kids are too young to be considering the risk of AIDS, you can use the techniques described in this book to deal with other sensitive issues, such as sexuality, drugs, or smoking. (See our discussion of other benefits in Chapter 10.) Establishing trust early can help your kids to be more open and cooperative with you later, when they're a little older, on the issues of AIDS-proofing.

- **Every chapter is essential.** We urge you to read this book in its entirety. We know that some of you may judge some chapters less important than others. But every chapter will provide, if not specific exercises that you're able to use, then at least some general pointers that will help you with whatever techniques you may devise for your family's use. In reading every chapter, you still may not read one as thoroughly as another. For this reason, and because we, as educators, have found that some redundancy can be valuable, we often repeat important points in different chapters. This also tends to make each chapter relatively self-contained, allowing you to review material without having to do too much jumping around in the book.

• **Try not to panic.** The fact that you are reading this book is a clear sign that you are concerned about AIDS-proofing your kids and are considering the use of a behavioral approach. Progressive coaching and realistic practice, backed up with approval and reward, should see you through any discomfort that you and your family may experience. But you may find that some aspects of this program are intensely upsetting. You may conclude that, in spite of your best intentions, you can't imagine yourself carrying them out, or you may run into problems when you do try to carry them out. If this should occur, we urge you to enlist the aid of a behavioral professional to work through this book with you and your kids. Your local healthcare and professional organizations can put you in touch with behavioral psychologists, social workers, counselors, or nurses — the key word here is *behavioral*. Get help if AIDS-proofing becomes too stressful.

3

Breaking the Ice: Start Talking

It is likely that many of you have been searching for as much information on AIDS as you can possibly find. This book is not an AIDS fact book, it is a book on how to protect your kids from the disease. But in order to protect them you will need to know the basic facts about AIDS. We therefore suggest that before you begin discussing AIDS with your kids you review the facts about this disease in Chapter 9. That chapter provides a summary of current knowledge about the disease and its modes of transmission. Of course, scientists are continually uncovering new facts about AIDS and the Human Immunodeficiency Virus (HIV) that causes it, so we advise you to keep abreast of these developments. A list of organizations that you can contact for more information is located in the back of this book.

Once you've familiarized yourself with the facts about AIDS, you'll want to plan an effective strategy for discussing this information with your kids.

The threat that AIDS poses to kids is probably not at the

top of your household's list of popular topics of conversation. AIDS is unpleasant to think about in its own right; the idea that your kids may need protection from this cruel disease is particularly disturbing. In addition, many parents don't like to acknowledge their kids' emerging sexuality, let alone the possibility that their kids may already be having sexual relations. So it won't be surprising if you find the prospect of discussing this issue with your kids very unpleasant — so unpleasant that you might prefer just to do nothing at all.

But the risks your kids face if you do nothing are simply too serious. That's why we're going to help you by having you apply the principles of progressive coaching. Progressive coaching along with realistic practice and generous amounts of approval and reward will provide you with a relatively painless way to approach your kids with the topics of AIDS and sex. First we'll have you build up your confidence by talking with another adult about AIDS and AIDS-proofing. Then we'll help you to find ways of introducing the topic to your kids with a minimum of discomfort for both of you. Finally we'll discuss how to gradually encourage your kids actively and constructively to discuss AIDS and AIDS-proofing with you.

TALK ABOUT AIDS WITH
ANOTHER ADULT FIRST

Talking about sex and AIDS with another adult will probably be a little easier for you than discussing it with your kids. Choose someone you find easy to talk to about sensitive topics. It might be your spouse or partner, or a close friend or relative. For simplicity's sake, we'll refer to your easy-to-talk-to adult as your "spouse."

We're going to have you apply progressive coaching to your conversations with your spouse. This will give you a chance to practice this technique before you apply the same principles with your kids. In addition, it will help minimize any discomfort you and your spouse might have in talking to each other about AIDS.

Remember the essentials of progressive coaching: start small, progress gradually, and readjust expectations when necessary. And be sure to maximize your use of praise and other positive reactions.

Here's how to proceed: Prepare a list of topics related to the broad theme of teenage sex and AIDS. Your list should start with a topic that you'd expect to cause you and your spouse the least discomfort, then progress step-by-step through increasingly difficult topics, and end with the topic of AIDS as a threat to your kids and what you can do to protect them. This is likely the subject you expect to be the most unpleasant to discuss. Progressing in this gradual manner will make you more and more comfortable discussing sensitive topics and will increase your confidence for your ultimate task of AIDS-proofing your kids.

To give you a concrete illustration of how to employ progressive coaching to "break the ice" with your spouse, we'll work step-by-step through our own list of topics. The details and order of your topics may differ from ours; what is important is that you start easy, progress in small steps, and, if necessary, back up when you encounter difficulties.

1. **Start easy.** Talking about your kids' dating is related to the topic of AIDS and teen sex, but is unlikely to cause you or your spouse much embarrassment, so we've placed it at the top of our list. Some specific questions you might discuss on this subject are:
   • How often do your kids go out on dates?
   • Does dating seem to be important to them?

- Have they been dating more often recently?
- Do they do more dating than you're happy with?
- Are they dating many different kids or only one or two? How do you both feel about this?
- How does their dating remind you of your own experiences at your kids' ages? Have the "rules" changed? Is this an improvement, in your opinion?

2. **Progress gradually to a slightly more difficult topic:** Are your kids seriously involved?
   - Do your kids have a "special someone" that they're seeing a lot of?
   - Are they spending more and more time with this boyfriend or girlfriend, to the exclusion of their other friends?
   - Are most of your kids' friends "coupled" these days? How do you both feel about this?
   - Are you seeing lots of public hand-holding and kissing between boyfriends and girlfriends?
   - Do your kids seem mature enough to be forming serious attachments?
   - Are their relationships getting in the way of their other activities?

   Some of these questions may provoke intense discussions. But what's more important than the particular conclusions you may come to is that having these discussions is helping you "break the ice."

3. **Gradually progress to an even more serious topic:** Your kids' sexual activity. If you haven't discussed this topic yet, you should by now feel a bit easier about doing so. Some possible questions for you to discuss are:

- Have you found sexually oriented magazines in your kids' rooms?
- Have you overheard your kids talking to their friends about sex?
- What seems to be their attitude toward sex?
- Have you noticed them doing some heavy-duty petting, perhaps before getting out of the car after a date?
- Do you think your kids are old enough to be having sex?
- Do you think they are having sex?
- Do you think that their friends are having sex?
- Do you think that your kids and their friends have purchased condoms?

Once again, your answers to these questions — and often you won't even know the answers — are less important than the fact that you are gradually progressing to increasingly touchy issues with your spouse. You're on the road to making AIDS-proofing a legitimate family matter.

4. **Now progress to a more difficult topic:** AIDS. You haven't been looking forward to this topic, but you're now much better prepared to discuss it. Review the medical information provided in Chapter 9. Get some pamphlets on AIDS from your doctor or public health office or from one of the organizations listed in the back of this book. Encourage your spouse to look over this material. If either of you find this material disturbing, apply the principle of progressive coaching by discussing the less-threatening material first.

   - You may find it easier to introduce the subject in a relatively impersonal manner by considering some of the more technical facts about the disease: the AIDS virus

(HIV), how it affects the immune system, the stages of AIDS, and some of the facts about the relative incidence of AIDS in different parts of the world.

- You may wish next to talk about some of the facts and concerns about AIDS that you've encountered in the media, perhaps including news reports of HIV infection in your community or notable figures who have contracted the disease.
- You should now be prepared to discuss how HIV is transmitted and the kinds of activities that put people at risk.

5. **You've broken the ice with your spouse.** You're now ready to face the most disturbing issue of all: Your kids could get AIDS. What are your responsibilities as a parent? You can and must try to protect your kids from AIDS.

We've taken you through a series of steps designed to make it easier for you to discuss AIDS and AIDS-proofing with your spouse. As we suggested earlier, the details aren't etched in stone; your own list may consist of somewhat different topics, and you may decide to progress through them in a different order. Only you can judge what is best for you and your situation. You must also judge how quickly to proceed from one subject to the next. Some of you may have one long discussion that covers your entire list. Others may feel more comfortable proceeding slowly, perhaps covering only one subject in each discussion, or even talking about the same subject several times before you're ready to progress further.

Keep the following points in mind as you proceed through your list:

- **Be flexible.** Be prepared to make changes in the list and in your own expectations at any time; you won't really know how you and your spouse will react until you start talking together. And take advantage of articles and television programs on AIDS and safer sex; they can provide a handy opening for a discussion with your spouse.

- **Take your time.** Follow a pace that minimizes your discomfort, raising more embarrassing or disturbing topics only as you feel better prepared to do so.

- **Be sensitive to your spouse.** Give your spouse lots of support as you both attempt to overcome your initial discomfort and embarrassment. Give lots of praise and approval for efforts made. Acknowledge your own discomfort — you may both feel more at ease admitting your apprehension than trying to hide it. And always be prepared to readjust your expectations; if a new topic is making you or your spouse too uncomfortable, go back to an earlier one that was less distressing. Watch for times when your spouse seems a bit more relaxed or when a good opening for the topic happens to present itself.

- **Don't forget humor.** A little bit of humor is never out of place. Welcome a joking or witty remark; it helps to relieve tension and can make a serious topic easier to discuss.

Remember that the more time you and your spouse can spend talking about anything related to AIDS, the more at ease you'll feel with the subject. Discomfort often decreases with greater exposure. The more comfortable you and your spouse become talking to each other, the easier you'll find it to discuss AIDS and AIDS-proofing with your kids.

If you should find, in spite of your best efforts, that your spouse is still unwilling or unable to cooperate with you, then you'll either have to approach someone else or take sole responsibility for AIDS-proofing in your home. Naturally, it would be better to make this a family effort, but not if it means jeopardizing the success of the entire venture.

When you and your spouse both feel ready to begin AIDS-proofing your kids, the two of you should read through this book together and discuss your reactions. Consider which suggestions you are or are not prepared to follow, where and how you think you should begin, and, in general, how you can best put these ideas into practice in your own circumstances.

Of course, your first step in AIDS-proofing your kids is to broach the subject of AIDS with them. The rest of this chapter will provide you with some specific suggestions for doing this.

Read over these suggestions with your spouse and consider, in detail, how you can best apply them in your home. Try them out on each other. Anticipate how your kids might react and, with our suggestions in mind, plan and practice how you might best respond. Work on your "delivery" a bit; try to make it and yourselves as relaxed as possible. Most important, always be constructive and positive with each other, *never critical.* You want these early steps in AIDS-proofing to be as pleasant as possible. Otherwise you might decide to drop the entire project. For your kids' sake, it's crucial that you avoid criticism and negativity throughout this and every other stage in your AIDS-proofing campaign.

GETTING YOUR KIDS TO LISTEN TO YOU

Using progressive coaching, you can gradually introduce the subject of AIDS to your kids with a minimum of discomfort for all concerned. We'll outline the steps you can follow; feel free to alter or add to them.

1. **Let your kids see materials on AIDS in your house.** Leave some of your pamphlets on AIDS lying around the house where your kids will see them. Let them notice you and your spouse reading this book. Leave it lying around so they can look at it. Leave the most provocative topics showing, to help attract your kids' attention. It's a small first step, and there's no guarantee they'll actually read anything you leave out for them, but it could help to introduce the topic of AIDS in a low-key way.

2. **Let your kids overhear you talking about AIDS.** Start making brief comments about AIDS to your spouse when your kids are barely within hearing range. Then progress gradually to very brief comments about it when they're in the same room or seated around the table with you. Your comments in the presence of your kids might gradually progress from a discussion of the more technical aspects of the AIDS virus and symptoms to the sexual aspects of AIDS transmission. As you "raise the ante" little by little, each step will make all of you a little more comfortable with the topic and make it more likely that you'll all be better prepared for your next step.

3. **Have your kids listen as you talk to them about AIDS.** Start addressing your remarks about AIDS directly to your kids. Once again, the principle of progressive coaching

dictates that you do this in a gradual fashion, beginning with comments that will be least likely to provoke a negative reaction and progressing step-by-step through more and more threatening material. You might start by making a remark about how many references to AIDS you've noticed in the media or about the number of pamphlets on AIDS that you've seen in medical offices. These remarks could be made "in passing," in a manner that suggests you're not expecting a reply. Next you could mention your own concern about AIDS and how you purchased this book because of that concern. You could gradually mention a few facts about AIDS that you've read in the medical chapter. Your next step would be to refer to some of the facts about AIDS that may have more direct implications for your kids themselves, such as the fact that public-health officials are concerned about teenagers who have unprotected sex, particularly with multiple partners.

Throughout this process of progressive coaching, be sure that you and your spouse provide each other with lots of encouragement for each little bit of progress. Praise each other for persisting in spite of discomfort and compliment each other for work well done. Let your kids notice this mutual support between you and your spouse. Remarks such as "I sure agree with your mom on that!" or "Dad's right about that!" will keep up your own motivation as well as making it clear to your kids that both you and your spouse share the same concerns about AIDS. Remember, you and your spouse may find these first stages rather uncomfortable. The more visible support you can give each other, the easier you'll find it to persevere. Soon, both you and your kids will feel more comfortable having AIDS as a topic of family conversation in your home.

GETTING YOUR KIDS TO TALK
TO YOU ABOUT AIDS

During this process of getting your kids used to hearing AIDS discussed in your house, you'll be waiting for them to respond to you in some way. How you should react to them when they do respond, and how you might prod them to respond if they don't, is the subject of the following section.

Don't expect too much in the beginning. Whatever first prompts a response from your kids, whether it's one of the pamphlets you've left around the house or one of the remarks about AIDS you've tossed at them, the most important thing to remember is to be prepared to react positively. And, as we've emphasized, progressive coaching means being satisfied initially with, and thus demonstrating approval for, even minimal responses from your kids. So, initially, keep your expectations low.

You may have to be satisfied at first with little more than "Yeah, I know" or "Yeah, I've heard about that" or even a grunt that merely acknowledges that they heard what you said. Find a way to react in a positive manner. A friendly remark such as "There sure are a lot of things to worry about, aren't there" or "I guess we were lucky when I was a kid; we didn't have to deal with things like AIDS" should be fine, perhaps accompanied by a warm pat on the back. Try to use a tone which suggests that you're genuinely pleased with even these very brief exchanges. Your kids should not feel pressured to respond in much greater detail, at least not at this stage.

When your kids respond in a slightly more constructive manner, offering you some small nugget of information about their own experience, knowledge, or concerns, be grateful for it. Do everything you can to make them feel that you really appreciate their contribution, no matter how small it may seem. Your sincere "That's interesting to hear" or "I'm glad you're telling me that" may not get your kids immediately to talk their hearts out to you, but it may encourage them to be more comfortable talking with you the next time, or the next. And, if it doesn't make you too uncomfortable, be open with them about your own feelings. If AIDS scares you to death, be willing to tell your kids, openly and honestly. Your candor may encourage theirs.

You may not like what you hear. Your problem may not be getting your kids to start responding to your comments about AIDS; your problem may be dealing with the way in which they reply. There are a number of problems that might occur when your kids begin responding to you, and you should be prepared for them:

Problem #1:
What if progressive coaching makes my kids suspicious?

At some point in your attempt to get your kids talking about AIDS, they may think they "smell a rat." They might throw an accusation at you, such as "Come on, Mom, is this just your way of finding out if I'm sleeping with anyone?" or "Dad, I wish you'd stop beating around the bush and just ask me whether I'm having sex or not. Isn't that what all this is about?"

Solution:
Be perfectly honest with them.
- Tell them that you do want to discuss a number of things with them, when they're ready to, and that the possibility that they're having sex is one of them.

- Explain that you and your spouse are concerned about the threat of AIDS and that you've been trying to bring up the subject as gently and gradually as possible.
- Assure them that you're not out to criticize or find fault with them. In fact, you want to work cooperatively with them to help protect them from AIDS. Who knows? You may find, to your pleasant surprise, that your kids are more prepared to sit down and discuss sex and AIDS with you than you anticipated. Perhaps they won't need much progressive coaching at all.

This is a good opportunity for us to clear up a misconception you may have about progressive coaching. You may have thought that progressive coaching is designed to conceal your real intentions from your kids. This is not true; if it were, we would certainly not have encouraged you to leave this book around where your kids could examine it and find out what progressive coaching is all about. You may have assumed that progressive coaching can work only if your kids don't know what you are planning to do. This is also not true; your kids may require progressive coaching whether or not they know what your intentions are. To illustrate the point, take the example of teaching swimming to a child who is afraid of deep water. You may have had this experience with your own children. You didn't hide your intention to teach them to swim in deep water, nor did you take your children too seriously when they insisted that they'd never be able to venture into the deep end of the pool. You probably got them used to standing, then floating, then paddling around in the shallow end of the pool before gradually progressing into deeper and deeper water. You were using progressive coaching.

Problem #2:
What if my kids are rude?

Your kids might throw out a smart-aleck remark such as "Hey, Dad. Mom seemed to be happy to listen to you talk about this stuff; why don't you pick on her again?" Be careful not to fly off the handle with them, even if they deserve it. Bear in mind that the whole topic of sex is probably a very uncomfortable one for your kids. It's not unreasonable for them to fear that anything they say on the subject may bring on criticisms or restrictions from you. Therefore, do not be surprised if they try to avoid the topic entirely by being rude.

Your job is to convince your kids that it is safe for them to discuss these issues with you. They'll only come to believe this if discussions on these subjects are as free from conflict and discomfort as you can possibly make them. The last thing you want to do is to make your kids more reluctant than they already are to talk to you about AIDS and sex. This is why you must do everything you can to avoid strife.

Solution:
Stay calm.

- Just try to ignore their lack of civility and as calmly as possible bring your attempt at discussion to a close.
- Readjust your expectations. The next time you raise the subject with them, go back to an earlier step that proved less troublesome.

Problem #3:
Suppose they're too rude to ignore?

Your kids might make a remark such as "Ah, come on, get off my back. I don't have to listen to this." They might even walk out of the room.

Solution:

Stay in control.

You certainly don't want to encourage this kind of behavior, but you must resist any impulse to come down heavily on your kids for it.

- Make a contract, such as, "When I raise the subject of AIDS in the house, I expect you to be polite. I'm willing to go so far as to give you the car next Saturday night or give you some money for pizza with your friends if you'll cooperate."

- Notice that you're promising your kids something positive for acting in desirable ways; you're not threatening them with punishment for acting in undesirable ways. Progressive coaching must always be accompanied by approval and reward, not punishment and conflict. If your AIDS-proofing project starts out on the wrong foot, it could put the whole program in jeopardy.

You may not like responding to your kids' offensive behavior by giving them incentives to behave properly. But you really have no choice — not if you are serious about encouraging your kids to start discussing AIDS with you.

Problem #4:

What if their replies reveal a serious ignorance about AIDS?

"Hey, I'm not worried about AIDS," they might say. "None of my friends could possibly have AIDS." This may not be the kind of response you are looking for, but it is a start! They didn't leave. And they are *talking* to you about AIDS.

Solution:
Have patience.

Later, after you've gradually increased your kids' confidence about sharing their reactions with you, however misinformed they may be, you'll have plenty of opportunities to gradually change their attitudes. Right now, you don't want them to regret being honest with you.

- Show appreciation.
- Tell them you're interested in what they have to say, before firmly but gently indicating your disagreement.
- Ask them to read Chapter 9 or some other appropriate material on AIDS so they can get more information on the subject.
- Most importantly, add more incentives, if necessary, to get them to do so.

Problem #5:
What if my kids don't respond to me at all?

If the AIDS pamphlets that you've been leaving around the house and the remarks you've made on the subject have not prompted a reply from your kids, you'll have to find more active ways to encourage them to start talking.

Solution:
Encourage them.

- You may be able to encourage them to respond by giving them some obvious openings to do so. Phrases such as "Did you know that (fact about AIDS)?" or "Have you heard about (fact about AIDS)?" might prompt them to say something.
- If subtle approaches don't evoke some active comments from your kids, consider a more direct approach. Try

asking them some questions, avoiding anything too personal at this stage. For example, if your kids are taking a sex-education class at school, you might ask, "Has AIDS been talked about in your health class yet? What did you and your friends think?" Or you could ask them if they've noticed anything about AIDS in the school paper or on television.

- Don't forget to react positively to their first responses and to be careful to avoid any questions that might make your kids feel defensive or embarrassed. Questioning them about their sexual experience, for example, should probably wait until later. Bring up this subject after you and your spouse have had some longer discussions with your kids about AIDS and their need to protect themselves from it. One springboard to such a discussion might be to ask them to look over Chapter 1 in this book, perhaps with you by their side, and to discuss with you their reactions to it. Later you can talk to your kids about some of the medical facts in Chapter 9 on AIDS and how the AIDS virus is transmitted. You will then have an easier time involving your children in the development of an AIDS-proofing plan for the whole family.

You don't need to plan all these exchanges in advance. In fact, spontaneous but well-timed remarks may prove particularly effective in breaking the ice with your kids. Also, the media may be of considerable help here. Ads for condoms are beginning to surface in magazines and even on television. AIDS has become a more commonplace topic on many soap operas. Even family-type sitcoms are beginning to introduce episodes dedicated to the topics of safer sex and AIDS. Check the summaries for upcoming shows in your television listings and note any programs that will be dealing with these topics. Watch these programs with your kids. Share in their reactions. When the opportunity arises to ask them about their opinions and to probe some of the issues raised in the shows, seize it! These spontaneous exchanges may prove more fruitful than many carefully planned, formal discussions.

Remember, your whole purpose is ultimately to make your kids willing to discuss highly sensitive, personal issues with you — issues that most kids don't talk to their parents about. In the chapters that follow, we give you all the advice we can so that you'll be able to deal with these issues comfortably and effectively. Getting you and your kids more relaxed in these first discussions of AIDS will provide a good foundation for what is to follow.

PART II

Teaching Safer Sex

4

Condoms:
Making Your Kids Experts

If your kids engage in sexual intercourse, they must use condoms. Review the medical material in Chapter 9 so that you understand why the use of condoms is so critical. But your kids won't be protected by simply being told about condoms or by simply being told of their necessity for safer sex. As we saw in Chapter 1, many kids are aware of the necessity for condoms but still don't use them. Nor will it be enough for your kids to use condoms occasionally. They must use them *always*. Your kids must learn to make it a habit to use condoms and to use them effectively. It is best if they learn how to use them effectively before they have their first full act of intercourse. For this to be ensured, your kids will have to learn and practice everything that's involved in using condoms, so that they will be able to do so with complete ease and confidence. You will need to provide lots of help and support during this entire process to ensure that it is made easy and painless for your kids.

The efficient application of condoms is critical for both

partners during sex, and thus it is a skill to be learned by both your sons and your daughters! You may be tempted to think that this skill is for boys only. But consider for a moment that a daughter who can't buy condoms, can't apply condoms, can't insist on condom protection, and won't carry her own condoms is at risk of contracting AIDS when she is faced with a fumbling or uncooperative boyfriend who may or may not be infected.

As we said earlier, mastering safer sex is no different from mastering any other skill. Behavior that is to occur correctly and efficiently must be learned well enough to become a habit. This applies to skilled athletes, musicians, and anyone else who must be prepared to do the right thing at the right time. We all acquire and polish our skills through practice, ideally under conditions as close as possible to the "real thing." This same advice goes for your kids when they are learning to use condoms.

You've probably noticed how much instruction it took before you could count on your kids to help around the house, to speak politely, or just to hang up their clothes. It likely took more than simply asking to get your kids to do these things consistently. It took some repeated coaching. You'll have to do the same thing in tackling this more difficult problem of AIDS-proofing your kids. We'll make you a better teacher so you can do this effectively.

For you to be able to count on your kids using condoms habitually and properly, you'll have to coach them in a number of skills:

- **Talking about condoms.** Unless you can bring up the role of condoms for safer sex and discuss it with your kids, it may be difficult to teach them the actual skills of condom use.

- **Purchasing condoms.** Your kids will have to learn to be their own suppliers. They're unlikely to come to you when they need them, thus advertising their every sexual expectation.

- **Effectively putting condoms on.** Your kids will have to learn how to apply condoms comfortably and sensually and in such a way that the condoms won't burst, slip off, or otherwise fail to protect them.

- **Asserting their requirement that sex be safe.** Your kids must learn to insist that a condom be applied and be applied in a timely way, even when their sexual partner has a strong preference not to use one.

- **Reliably carrying condoms with them.** Your kids can't use condoms if they don't have them at hand. They're unlikely to dash out to the all-night pharmacy when in the heat of passion.

Let's get started. Let's get your kids talking to you about condoms. They may not be eager to do this, so we'll suggest some possible approaches to take. Of course, we realize that you may have to alter the details to suit your situation or to bypass certain steps that are unnecessary. Be careful, though; don't try to progress too quickly and ignore important considerations.

TALKING ABOUT CONDOMS

If your kids are reluctant to talk to you about condoms, as many probably will be, progressive coaching will help. In progressive coaching, as we said in Chapter 2, you must have some idea of the minimal behavior you can expect from your kids. In this case, that involves talking about condoms.

Unless your kids are extremely compliant and will listen to and discuss anything you have to say, begin slowly with a very casual mention of condoms. The recent appearance of ads on television or in magazines could provide the context. In addition casual comments could be made during times in which you and your kids are together and involved in other activities. For example, you could turn to your spouse to discuss some aspect of condoms: their price, or, in a lighter way, their new colors, shapes, and sizes. Will your kids pick up on this and contribute with a comment or with some good-natured laughter? Be careful to notice their reactions and respond to them. Any reaction they have, short of silence or disgust, should be responded to in a positive way, such as with a nod or a good-natured laugh.

Whatever your starting point, make sure you keep the conversation brief and low-key at first, using all the ease and casualness you can muster. You'll have time on later occasions gradually to increase the length and seriousness of your discussions.

If your kids don't immediately react in a receptive way, pull back and broach the topic again at another time. If they react in disgust or with extreme negativity to just the mere mention of condoms, then it may be time to consider "upping the ante." Make privileges dependent on just minimal, passive attention on their part. For example: "Hey, if you want the car tonight, then please listen to me for a few moments. You don't have to say anything, just listen."

Progressive coaching demands beginning at a point at which success is most likely to occur. Keep your initial expectations for your kids low and keep your sensitivity to their reactions high. At first you may have to be satisfied with just their passive listening. But take heart. If you slowly increase your daily demands on them for conversation, the topic can become one of little stress, some humor, and much benefit for your future AIDS-proofing efforts.

Your goal so far is just to be able to discuss comfortably the general necessity of condoms for safer sex and to have your kids agree that purchasing condoms is an important start to AIDS-proofing their lives.

GETTING YOUR KIDS TO BUY CONDOMS

Purchasing condoms is an essential and relatively easy first step for your kids to take in practicing safer sex. You may be tempted, however, to bypass this step and simply offer to supply them yourself. Although such intentions are admirable, keep in mind that your kids' best source for condoms is a store. Your kids won't want to announce their every move or romantic intention to you by having to ask you for a condom. Their desire for some privacy could mean that just that one time, when they need condoms the most, they won't have them. This is not a comforting thought. Knowing that they'll find it easy to get condoms on their own, whenever needed, is a lot more assuring.

If your kids already have some condoms, don't necessarily bypass this "learning-to-purchase" step. They may have been given a condom by a friend, or they may have used one of the vending machines in public restrooms. In either case, these sources are not readily available in the evening just before a date, whereas drug stores are. And, although your kids may have acquired a condom, they have not demonstrated to you that they're comfortable with buying them.

Failing to be comfortable in this step could later mean failing to be protected.

If your kids are at all uneasy about buying condoms — if they're uncomfortable about reaching for them on a drug-store shelf or asking a pharmacist for them and then taking them to a cashier, you'll have to help them. Sometimes, as we mentioned earlier, progressive coaching is unnecessary if simply offering a highly valued reward for doing a desired behavior will work. Thus, for some of you, simply promising your kids the use of the family car, the receipt of a bonus in their allowance, or free access to their choice of an evening's television programs in return for their "proof of purchase" of a package of condoms may be all that's necessary. Repeated practice will then help your kids become quite confident and self-assured about purchasing them. You must be the judge here as to whether this is workable in your situation. If so, it can be a terrific time-saver; if not, then progressive coaching is your alternative.

Progressive coaching must begin with an action your kids find easy and acceptable to do.

- Start by having them simply walk into a store, along with you if they need to, and locate the shelf where condoms are displayed. Their success, however small it may seem, must be praised or otherwise rewarded in some agreed-upon way.

- On the same or subsequent day, progress to a cursory reading of the labels to discover what brands and prices are involved. Don't forget to provide, at inconspicuous times, the praise or tangible rewards that you have promised as a part of this "game." The pay-off shouldn't be made until they display proof of their "window shopping" by showing some knowledge about local brands and prices.

- The actual purchasing of condoms is the final task and is a major step toward your kids' independent practice of safer sex. This crucial step requires some sensitivity on the part of the store personnel. Make the pharmacist or sales clerk aware of what you're doing with your kids so as to avoid any embarrassment at the time of purchase. Nothing could be more harmful to your kids' efforts than the slightest hint of judgment or amusement from the clerk. It would be a shame for the occasion to be marred by a shout to a stock boy for a price, a hesitation, a doubtful glance, a casual remark, or a humorous comment. This moment is critical! A few thoughts beforehand on how you can ensure your kid's success could literally be a lifesaver.

PUTTING CONDOMS ON EFFECTIVELY

Condoms purchased are not necessarily condoms used! The effective application of condoms by your kids will likely require some progressive coaching. What is meant by "effective application" is your kids' skill at effortlessly unwrapping a condom and applying it quickly, with a minimum of fuss and fumbling. Lack of skill in putting on condoms can be a source of embarrassment and a disruption of ongoing pleasures. In both cases, clumsiness will breed disuse. The development and practice of these skills is not a minor consideration, as many adults are incompetent with condoms as well.

To begin training effective condom application, you should use the following suggestions:

- Effectiveness in applying condoms can be easily practiced by the use of props such as broom handles, cucumbers, or other penis-shaped items. Quickly and efficiently unrolling condoms onto such hard items is an easy place to start.

- Practicing condom application in the form of a game, with "time-trials" and prizes or humorous awards, could help to prevent uneasiness or resistance.

- The next and more demanding skill your kids need to learn is how to unroll the condom onto a semierect penis. Practice should be encouraged on a sausage or an overripe, rather flaccid carrot as a means of simulating a partially erect penis. Your kids must learn how to apply a condom so that fingernails don't damage the delicate latex and do not excessively bend or pinch what will ultimately be a real penis. Both boys and girls should become "experts" at this.

- Your son's skill can be further improved by encouraging him to try on a condom during masturbation. (See Chapter 8 for more discussion of masturbation.) This will provide the most realistic condition, short of intercourse, for condom use. Trying out a condom during masturbation will also teach your son what to do with a used condom: having a tissue ready for wrapping it up. This is a lesson best learned now rather than after the delicate moments of lovemaking.

There are some problems frequently associated with using condoms. It is vital for you and your kids to know about these problems so they can be overcome:

Problem #1:
Condoms slip off.

Partially rolled-on condoms are more likely to come off during intercourse, but fully rolled-on condoms are more apt to get caught in pubic hairs.

Solution:

For boys, keep the pubic hairs at the base of the penis trimmed. For boys and girls alike, encircle the penis with thumb and forefinger so as to push the hairs back, away from the unrolling condom. For girls, take the time needed for a careful and full unrolling, so as to avoid trapping pubic hairs and to make the whole experience more sensual.

Problem #2:
Condoms burst.

A condom fitting tightly against the end of the penis is more likely to burst or to spread semen back over the penis, which might cause the condom to slip off during the last thrusts of intercourse.

Solution:

Pinch the end of the condom between the thumb and forefinger just at the start of unrolling. This will provide a small, airless "pocket" at the end of the condom. Condoms with "tips" or built-in pockets should be treated in exactly the same way. This pocket can receive the semen and retain it while also providing a reserve of condom material to allow for the stretching needed during the thrusts of intercourse. Slipping and bursting will be less likely, and so will the transmission of HIV.

Problem #3:
Condoms pinch.

Unrolling a condom on a somewhat soft or flaccid penis is more likely to pinch the skin and discourage further use. An initial erection may start to fade as the mechanics of condom application begin.

Solution:

Girls can fondle and excite the penis into full erection. Boys can try some masturbation to achieve or restore full erection. Trying to unroll a condom on a soft penis is painful and risky. Don't let your kids think otherwise.

IMPORTANT CONDOM TIPS TO REMEMBER

- Use only latex condoms — natural or lambskin condoms let HIV pass through them.
- Condoms vary; finding a comfortable condom may increase your partners willingness to use them.
- The condom must be put on before penetration, because the virus can be present in pre-ejaculatory fluid.
- If you need additional lubrication for vaginal or anal intercourse, use only a water-based, water-soluble lubricant, such as K-Y® jelly, that does not damage latex. Lubricants containing alcohol, mineral or vegetable oils, or petroleum jelly can cause condoms to deteriorate quickly and to break.
- To further reduce the risk of breakage, try extra-strength or ribbed condoms, or use two at once.

- Use unlubricated condoms for oral sex.
- No penis is too big or too small for a condom — snug-fit condoms are available for smaller penises.
- Do not store condoms in a warm place. Heat can weaken the material and cause holes or tears in the condom during sex.
- Latex condoms may provide greater protection when used with a spermicide, such as nonoxynol-9 (a substance that has been shown to kill the AIDS virus [HIV] in laboratory tests). Spermicides are contained in contraceptive (birth-control) foams, in some lubricants, and in some lubricated condoms. Never use a spermicide alone instead of a condom.
- Always use a new condom. When a used condom is reapplied it can bring old semen and vaginal fluids into contact with the penis and vagina, thereby counteracting its protection. Also, a condom is more likely to break or slip off with multiple use. *Never* use the same condom more than once.

Courtesy of the American College Health Association and the American Red Cross

You may be surprised to read that condoms are mistakenly used more than once by some people. This dangerous mistake is often made by kids. It is important that you know the reasons why this occurs and what alternatives you can suggest:

Reason#1:
It seems to feel better.
Some guys say that the previous ejaculation makes the condom slippery on the inside and that this is a real "turn-on" for him in subsequent intercourse.

Solution:

A dab of a water-based lubricant on just the tip of the penis before putting the condom on can provide these same sensations. Let your kids know this little "secret."

Reason #2:
It seems easier.

Putting on another condom carries with it the same risks of fumbling, embarrassment, and distraction as putting the first one on.

Solution:

Practice and overlearn, outside of a sexual situation, all the skills mentioned in this chapter. The solution is partly up to you.

Reason #3:
It's cheaper.

Condoms are expensive for many kids. Kids may be tempted to make one condom serve the purpose of two or more when they can't afford them.

Solution:

Underwrite their expenses. Create a "condom account," but do it at arm's length. Don't make them come to you for the money just before they go out on their date; that's advertising that they can likely do without. Here is another reason why daughters must carry condoms as well. By purchasing condoms, they help to underwrite the expenses of their partner as a contribution to safer sex. Latex condoms are less costly than the more exotic, expensive "skins." Latex is more prone to break, but it is less likely to allow the HIV virus to pass through. In this case "cheaper" is better.

A condom used again is an unacceptable risk. Old, unused condoms are risky business too. Your kids should be advised to replace them periodically. According to *Consumer Reports* (March 1989), translucent or transparent packaging ages condoms faster; stickiness, discoloration, or drying out are the signs of deterioration. Consult your pharmacist; condoms have a limited "shelf life" of up to five years if stored in a cool, dark, dry place. It is unlikely that kids will use such a storage place. Replacement, however, can be an unwanted expense. Underwrite this expense. It's cheap insurance.

Your kids must learn to deal with all these problems in a manner skillful enough to avoid the embarrassment of fumbling and ineptness. Skillfulness guarantees a minimum of interference with ongoing pleasures, thus helping to ensure that condoms will continue to be used in the future. If kids aren't good at using condoms, they will stop using them. All that we know about human learning stands behind this warning.

TEACHING ASSERTIVENESS AND THE TIMELY USE OF CONDOMS

Assertiveness and timely use refers to your kids' interpersonal skill at successfully insisting on the use of a condom early enough in the act of sex to be undeterred by the heat of passion. Genital contact must not take place until a condom is in place. Keep in mind that this mandatory and timely use of condoms is important to both sexes, and it is thus a skill to be learned and practiced by both your sons and daughters.

The actual conditions in which condoms are used are private and away from parental involvement. You will not be there to help your kids be assertive and engage in timely use. Your kids can, nonetheless, learn these skills by practicing them under simulated, role-playing conditions. In a role-play, a parent or appropriately aged sibling can play the part of a careless sex partner who is trying to avoid the use of a condom by the more levelheaded sex partner. Your kids can be coached in how to deal with such difficulties. Keep in mind that the timely use of a condom means having it ready and putting it on before the level of passion rises to the point of throwing caution to the wind. Try remembering your first heated sexual encounters and the temptation to ignore precautions under these circumstances.

Before you can get down to the actual development of a role-play for your kids, they will have to clearly recognize the need for assertiveness and timeliness in using condoms. If your kids have not been sexually active up to now, they may have a hard time appreciating how, in the heat of passion, the detour to a condom may be distracting or how the boy, possibly in a higher state of arousal, may resist this detour or want to try some brief genital contact before putting on a condom. If your kids have already had the experience of sharing some of the passions of sex, they'll undoubtedly be reluctant to share the details of these moments with you. And yet this issue of assertiveness and timeliness must be discussed.

The painless approach to this problem involves progressive coaching. You'll have to start your discussion on assertiveness and timeliness in the use of condoms at a level that will cause little or no embarrassment.

By this point in your interactions with your kids, you'll already have some idea as to what type of discussion they will initially feel comfortable with. Try this "comfortable" level of discourse with them, as always, in a low-key and casual way. This may mean nothing more than mom dropping a brief, light-hearted comment about the single-minded pursuit of immediate pleasure by men in sexual situations. Or dad might make a light comment about how using condoms is like taking a shower with your raincoat on. Admittedly, such comments may reflect stereotypes or corny humor, but they're icebreakers nonetheless. Comments separated by minutes or days, depending on your reading of your kids' tolerances, can gradually escalate into sharing with them your own impatience or awkwardness in dealing with condoms at times of making love. You might briefly relate to them your earliest experiences, or those of friends, with the "ever-challenging condom." The key here is to be casual.

Once you have a starting point for discussion, you must increase the demands on the content of these brief conversations. Your goal is to be able to talk for longer periods about how difficult it can be to insist on safer sex and how awkward it would be to interrupt the impatient demands of passion to insist on the use of a condom. Take small steps, over days and weeks if necessary, and proceed at a comfortable pace for all.

But it's not sufficient for your kids just to agree that they might find it difficult to insist on using a condom. Nor will it be sufficient for your kids just to agree that a condom should be put on early in a sexual interaction, before passion takes over. Simply recognizing and agreeing to the existence of these problems is not learning how to deal with them. Role-plays will provide your kids with the opportunity to actually rehearse and practice being insistent and timely. It's in the role-play that they'll learn to assert their need to use a condom. And it's in the role-play that they'll learn to make this assertion early in a sexual encounter. For this reason, we urge you: *do not skip this step*, no matter how much assurance your kids give you that it's really not necessary, no matter how much assurance they give you that they understand what you're telling them. Knowing is not the same as doing!

Role-playing can involve completely scripted lines for the two roles of the levelheaded and careless sex partners. The script should be prepared by all of you and then given to each "actor" to modify so it fits his or her style and needs. Or each "actor" may improvise his or her own role, with your input to ensure accuracy. The choice depends on your judgment as to which style best suits your family.

Since several scenarios may likely be necessary to cover a variety of circumstances, more than one role-play should be developed. You must anticipate, with wisdom from your own experiences, the types of situations your kids may encounter.

The words your kids choose to use must be clear and concise, with no hints of uncertainty, yet the words must be gentle and caring ones that will not offend a real-life partner.

The effect that timely insistence might have on the feelings of "careless" partners must be considered. This is to avoid inciting a punishing or uncompromising reaction from them. Resistance by the "loved one" could produce guilt and subsequent giving-in to carelessness on the part of your kids. These are the nuances that must be included, as completely as possible, so that the role-plays will be the most helpful. You don't have to be a Hollywood writer; you're not out to get an Oscar. You have to recognize these very human reactions, discuss them, and try to build them into your role-plays.

Once your kids have learned, during the pretended sexual encounters, how to clearly and sensitively demand that a condom be used, they'll then need some practice at tenacity. No matter how clear and caring their demands, some partners may still refuse to comply. Your kids will need practice in un-bending but gentle insistence in the face of a more and more resistant partner. Several short role-plays can be developed in which the levelheaded partner is presented with an in-creasingly uncooperative, careless partner. By practicing such a series of short role-plays with your help and prompt-ing, your kids can painlessly and reliably learn to stand up for themselves.

You might include some final scripts in which the careless partner is as dominating and scornful as possible. Your son or daughter could face a lot of pressure in a real situation and must be well-prepared for it. They'll also have to be prepared for the careless partner who simply and finally refuses to use a condom. Your son's or daughter's only option then will be to end the encounter without sexual intercourse. The words for doing this must be well-chosen and rehearsed, and they must fit your kids' style of speech so that they'll feel natural and comfortable saying them.

As your kids develop and rehearse these role-plays with you, remember to keep true to the idea of progressive coach-ing. Being assertive may not come easily or naturally to them; they may need to learn it gradually. Work with small steps and be generous in your approval for your kids' small-est accomplishments. No matter how insufficient these ac-complishments may initially seem, this is the effective way to develop behavior.

An initial role-play could have a script not too different from the one presented below, but our script is just a starting point for you. You'll have to develop scripts that are "home-grown," containing the words and phrases your kids might actually use. Help them develop short, firm statements. Have them avoid justification or argument; this only invites counterarguments. Throughout the scripts you develop together, your kids' message must always be straightforward and simple: No sex without safety!

Boy Resisting Girl's Application of Condom

BOY: What are you doing?

GIRL: I'm getting out a condom.

BOY: What! You've got to be kidding.

GIRL: (*Note: Girl does not get defensive.*) No, I'm serious.

BOY: Hey, I'm not going to use one of those things.

GIRL: I don't want to have sex without protection.

BOY: I thought you were on the Pill . . . all the girls are, you know . . . why aren't you?

GIRL: (*Note: Girl avoids getting into the side-issue of the Pill.*) Using this condom will make things safe for both of us. I don't want either of us to risk getting AIDS.

BOY: Look, I don't have AIDS and I don't think you do either, so let's stop all this. This is dumb!

GIRL: (*Note: Girl avoids an unanswerable issue and refuses to be sidetracked.*) You're right, we probably don't have AIDS, but I really don't think we should take risks.

BOY: (*With increasing frustration.*) You're really crazy, you know? None of my friends use condoms, and their girlfriends haven't gotten pregnant. And no one has gotten AIDS either!

GIRL: If we have sex, I want it to be with a condom. (***Note:*** *Notice that she doesn't try to contradict him. She remains calm but firm. Of course, she should practice another scenario in which she ends the sexual encounter; this must be coached as well.*)

Girl Resisting Boy's Application of a Condom

GIRL: What do you think you're doing?

BOY: I'm getting out a condom.

GIRL: Don't do that; I hate those things. And besides, I'm on the Pill.

BOY: (***Note:*** *Boy refuses to get sidetracked.*) You may be on the Pill, but this is to protect us both from AIDS.

GIRL: Oh, come on! Do you know anyone with AIDS? Don't be such a worrier!

BOY: (***Note:*** *Boy doesn't get defensive, but steadfastly and nicely asserts his wishes.*) I don't want us to take any chances. I'm sorry if you don't like it, but this is best for both of us.

GIRL: Look, I won't have sex with condoms.

BOY: I'm really sorry that you feel that way. I hope you'll change your mind sometime.

These are just two possible scripts. Don't feel you have to stick to them. Quite the contrary. The more your kids can use their own words to the same effect, the better. Also, you'll want all the ideas from them that you can get.

Other script variations might deal with a partner who is so aroused that he or she doesn't want to wait even a moment for intercourse. Of course, practicing rapid and effective application of a condom and keeping in mind the importance of early, timely use will also help your kids deal with this situation.

In Chapter 5 we discuss safe alternatives to intercourse. These options may provide additional approaches for your kids to pursue.

When several role-play scenarios have been developed, performed, and seem comfortable to your child, the key word becomes *practice*. You should attempt to make your role-playing as realistic as possible to encourage effective condom use in actual sexual encounters. Practicing these sensitive subjects will make them more habitual and therefore more likely to be used when needed. Role-playing that may seem easy for your kids to perform once or twice may likely be forgotten when the pressure is on, unless practice goes far beyond just a few token "rehearsals."

Practice of any skill can get boring, as we all know. The problem is no less with these intimate behaviors and, in addition, there will always be some degree of discomfort that will discourage practicing them.

To keep motivation high, you should be very generous with praise for your kids' continued practice. You'll likely also have to give your kids material incentives. There is little pleasure in the continued practicing of these social/sexual skills. The situation is no different for kids doing their school homework, practicing the piano, or developing other skills in preparation for adulthood. A common practice for parents is to provide material incentives to optimize learning. We strongly suggest that you do no less with these fragile social/sexual skills.

It's time to think again about what rewards your kids will work for. Consider the use of the family car for older kids; favorite foods and television programs; opportunities for parties and other social events; tickets to movies, sports, or other entertainments; and whatever other things your kids might identify as being worth receiving. This issue of AIDS prevention is too serious for you to be tightfisted with the family resources.

If the idea of giving rewards still makes you uncomfortable, remember that your kids will be earning their rewards. Their "job" is to role-play and rehearse lifesaving habits that are healthy, sensible, and will see them through the coming decades. This should, justifiably, make you feel like a concerned and actively involved parent.

TEACHING YOUR KIDS TO CARRY CONDOMS

You must decide together with your kids how they will carry condoms: in a wallet, purse, pocket, or some other means. Your kids should be encouraged to carry more than one condom at a time because of the extreme dangers of using a condom more than once. Some kids may try using a condom more than once due to their general ignorance of condom use. Multiple use of a condom is extremely risky behavior. They should carry two or more condoms with them at all times so that multiple use can be absolutely avoided.

Another important thing your kids may not know is that sexual encounters can occur under the most unlikely or unexpected circumstances. This means that condoms must be readily available in a "holder" that is almost constantly with them. Some clothing manufacturers are selling color-coordinated, designer condom holders. This may be a great idea for a coming birthday or holiday gift, as well as providing an initial opportunity to broach the subject with the pre-teens in your household.

It may be difficult to get your kids to actually carry condoms. Although some boys may be in social circles in which condoms are a mark of status, many kids may see them as a possible source of embarrassment. You can ease their anxieties by simply pointing out the high priority that should be given to safer sex. Helping your kids find a discreet way to carry condoms might also solve the problem. Although it is surely best for them to carry condoms on their person, giving them the only key to a locked glove compartment in the family car, so that others can't keep track of their use, may be well worth the inconvenience to you or your spouse. For carrying condoms on their person, change purses are suitable. Makeup compacts, cassette cases, picture or credit card holders, renovated for condom concealment, are other possibilities. Ask your kids for ideas. Let your imaginations soar. Organize a family write-in contest with suitable rewards for the best ideas. Reap the benefits of at least making these concerns easier to talk about and more acceptable to everyone. Failing these efforts, a simple contract with your kids may be necessary.

Contracting with your kids to carry condoms can be quite straightforward. If your praise and approval means a lot to them, then show it when you periodically ask them to show you that they have condoms with them. Of course, approval is given only if they have condoms with them when you check.

But be careful not to make the whole process seem like a police examination. One way to avoid this is to let your kids earn really important and valued incentives so that they have especially good reasons to approach you for a "checkup." With the continued use of really worthwhile incentives, at least until your kids can fully appreciate the importance of preparedness, they'll also be less likely to complain about not being trusted or about being treated like babies.

There's little purpose in dealing with the entire issue of condoms if you're not going to ensure that your kids are carrying them and will have them when they're needed. Be generous.

FOLLOW-UP!

The final test of your kids use of condoms, of course, is whether or not they will put them on in an effective and timely way under conditions of sexual intimacy. Even though you won't be there to see this, you should be willing to provide positive support and honest advice if your kids should confide in you as to their success, failure, or difficulties. Teasing or other potentially embarrassing reactions should be avoided at all cost. This is not the time to unilaterally express your possible concerns over moral issues relating to promiscuity, sex before marriage, and other valid considerations. This is the time to be considerate and caring and supportive in whatever ways you can. At this moment, to encourage their continuing openness with you, your self-control and measured reactions are extremely important.

5

Spread the Word:
Alternatives to Intercourse

Intercourse without effective use of a condom is unsafe. But you may not be prepared to teach your kids to use condoms effectively. Or you might feel that even if you did teach your kids properly, knowing your kids as you do, they would not reliably use condoms in all circumstances. If so, you should consider the following: The best defense your kids may have from AIDS, with the exception of abstaining from sex (which is discussed in the next chapter), is to have sex without intercourse. There are safer, alternative ways to enjoy sex with a partner.

Many people feel that sexual intercourse is the ultimate way to express one's caring and intimate feelings with a loved one. We don't disagree. But we do think that this generation of kids has to consider alternative practices, particularly when they may be active sexually, often with multiple partners, prior to marriage.

Because sexual transmission of AIDS occurs primarily through intercourse, alternative sexual practices offer a practical way to reduce the risk of infection. If your kids are to avoid intercourse, what are their alternatives? Will your kids be prepared to engage in them? Will they consider sexual alternatives as legitimate or as perversions? Will they be skilled enough in alternatives to satisfy both themselves and their partners? Only if both partners enjoy the sexual act will they be content not to have intercourse. It therefore is critical for your kids to become as knowledgeable as possible about pleasurable alternatives to intercourse before they find themselves in sexually demanding situations.

With this in mind, you should consider acquainting yourself, if you haven't already, with a variety of sexual alternatives. But you may have objections to the idea of sexual alternatives to intercourse. Some people have been taught that anything other than intercourse is unwholesome or "wrong." If this is the way you feel, it might help you to know that many counselors recommend a wide variety of sexual alternatives to their clients. They usually do this in order to bring new excitement and vitality to sexual relationships. This has nothing to do with safer sex, but the implication is clear: There are alternatives to intercourse that can be enjoyed as safer sex.

SEXUAL ALTERNATIVES TO INTERCOURSE AND HOW TO FIND THEM

A look through books and magazines with sexual themes will reveal a number of variations in approaches to sexual enjoyment. Choose those most acceptable to you. For example:

- Mutual masturbation with a partner
- Oral sex
- Nonorgasmic sexual play followed by masturbation to orgasm

We cannot guarantee that any of these alternatives is totally safe, therefore suitable precautions should always be taken when engaging in them. (See Chapter 9 for detailed precautions and suggestions.)

Other variations involving visual or mechanical aids to sexual enjoyment are also depicted and talked about in our culture.

Even so-called "readers' letters" in popular magazines, though likely fabricated or at least embellished by editors, depict many variations that are practiced in our culture.

In addition to popular publications, pamphlets such as the American College Health Association's "Safer Sex" and "Making Sex Safer" and the Canadian AIDS Society's "Safer Sex Guidelines" argue for the consideration of alternative sexual behaviors and provide information about the relative risk involved with these activities. These sources, listed at the end of Chapter 10, are worthy of your careful consideration.

A WORD OF CAUTION

Any sexual interaction with an infected person involves some degree of risk if it allows for the exchange of bodily fluids (semen, vaginal fluids, blood, urine, and even breast milk). For example, although saliva is not a good medium for transmitting HIV, sores or cuts in the mouth that allow blood to be transferred during "wet" kissing add significantly to the risk involved. Similarly, if your fingers contact semen or vaginal fluid, you would ordinarily be at little risk, but if there is an open sore on a finger, or even a hangnail, contact with an infected partner could significantly increase the risk of infection with HIV. A finger inserted into the vagina may tear the vaginal lining, greatly increasing the receptive partner's risk should unprotected intercourse follow. Unprotected oral sex may seem to be a less risky activity than unprotected intercourse, but the exact risk of HIV transmission through oral sex has not yet been defined, and the existence of any type of sore or cut in the mouth would significantly increase the risk involved. Mutual masturbation in which semen or vaginal fluids are brought into contact with the opening of the penis, rectum, or vagina is certainly not a low-risk activity.

Thus, it must be emphasized that low-risk activities may not necessarily be low risk and that low risk is not the same as no risk. Therefore, protection in the form of condoms, latex gloves, or other suitable protective devices should always be used with these alternatives to intercourse. Contact your local AIDS organization for advice. Moreover, as pointed out in Chapter 4, a condom is only as effective as the integrity of its material and the care and expertise of its user.

Mixing sex with alcohol or drugs is also a very risky practice. It increases the likelihood that caution, inhibitions, and safer sex will be abandoned in favor of much riskier sex practices.

SAFE BUT SEXY: SOME EXAMPLES

Each of the following activities can be highly erotic and is AIDS-safe, as long as there is no contact with the genitalia or anus and no exchange, direct or indirect, of bodily fluids. They can be practiced alone or followed by self-masturbation:

- Dry kissing
- Body-to-body rubbing
- Telephone sex
- Erotic films, videos, books, magazines
- Body licking and kissing
- Fantasy

- Erotic talk
- Massage/touch/caresses
- Erotic bathing or showering
- Unshared sex toys

PSYCHOLOGICAL AND MORAL ISSUES

As you consider these alternatives to sexual intercourse, you may conclude that some of them are less appropriate than others. You may have some concerns as to how psychologically healthy or morally acceptable they are. And you may hope for "expert" professional advice to help you.

Our position, and you may feel disappointed by it, is that nothing can replace your own values and instincts on these matters. We would prefer to have some definite answers for you. But the simple fact is that the "experts" — social scientists, health professionals, philosophers, and clerics — themselves have differences of opinion on these issues, and their public statements often appear to be a reflection of their own subjective opinion. To our knowledge there has been little scientific work that has reported data on the possible harm or, for that matter, benefit from practicing any of these sexual alternatives.

There is, however, much agreement on one issue. A preoccupation with sex to the exclusion of other social and interpersonal activities *is* likely to be "unhealthy." We are certainly not advocating unlimited sexual indulgence or promiscuity. Far from it! Also, we do not want you to ignore the many other problems of parenting by exclusive attention to the risks of AIDS, nor do we advocate that your interactions with your kids be dominated by discussions of AIDS, sex, and related matters. We are simply trying to help ensure that if your kids are involved in sexual activity, they do so with minimal risk.

ANYTHING GOES?

Although we feel that no "expert" is in a position to make general pronouncements about which sexual practices are right or wrong, we're not suggesting that no judgments at all be made. You may feel that some practices you have read about or seen depicted are degrading, exploitative, or otherwise questionable. Knowing your own kids, you may have some serious concerns about whether they or their potential sex partners are psychologically and emotionally prepared for some forms of intimacy. If your son or daughter is getting any type of therapeutic treatment, the professional involved may also have some concerns on this matter. Either your knowledge of your kids or your general values may lead you to reject certain sexual practices.

We think it's important to discuss your values and concerns with your kids. Share your ideas with them. Give them a chance to understand your reservations and to express and discuss their own emerging attitudes with you. As their parents, you have to be the ones to communicate gently and carefully the sexual options they have in avoiding the risks of intercourse. Do not count on books, magazines, videos, and other publications that consider sexual techniques to deal with these issues for you. The very existence of these sources gives implicit approval to the sexual variations that they illustrate or discuss. Unfortunately, kids don't usually examine this kind of material when their parents are around to offer advice. A lot of trust between you and your kids should make them more willing to consider the information in such materials with you. We hope that some of the recommendations in this book will help to develop or maintain this trust.

Ideally, you'll want to do more than just influence which alternatives to intercourse your kids will explore; you'll also want to help shape their attitudes toward these practices.

In some cases, depending on their age, your kids may already have some knowledge about alternative sexual practices. But you can't count on that knowledge being accurate. Many kids learn to regard alternative sexual practices as questionable perversions, or as unmanly or unwomanly, or as just not "cool." Attitudes like these will certainly not encourage your kids to adopt these practices.

For example:

- If your kids have the idea that masturbation is "dirty" or unhealthy, are they likely to consider such fondling of their partner or by their partner to be a perfectly acceptable AIDS-proof alternative to intercourse?

- Will they know enough to be able to masturbate each other effectively so that they'll both be satisfied enough not to have intercourse?

- After tiring of one alternative to intercourse, will they go on to experiment with other enjoyable alternatives? Or will they fear the judgmental label of promiscuity?

- Will they approach the subject of alternatives with the attitude that "it isn't cool" or with an open mind?

Clearly, we as parents have a very important role in shaping our kids' sexual attitudes and values and in combating less enlightened influences. Your caring adult input could put alternative sexual practices in a better and healthier perspective.

One such perspective is the one we've suggested here: Sexual variations that provide alternatives to unprotected or unreliably protected sexual intercourse are a means of reducing the risk of AIDS.

ARE ALL SEXUAL ALTERNATIVES
EQUALLY AIDS-SAFE?

The medical information in this book will allow you and your kids to evaluate the relative risks associated with different sexual practices. Additional information can be found in the many sources listed at the end of Chapter 10. As new medical information emerges you may have to reassess the risk associated with each sexual alternative. You'll need an ongoing and trusting relationship with your kids to do this. Much of what we're suggesting in this book is designed to help you establish this relationship or to keep you from undermining it as you and your kids together face the issue of AIDS.

DO SEXUAL ALTERNATIVES MAKE YOU BLUSH?

Many people and institutions in our culture believe that interpersonal sex implies intercourse. Some of them, as we've already mentioned, believe that intercourse is the only proper form of interpersonal sex. There are many taboos regarding alternative forms of sexual expression. For this reason, it won't be surprising if you and your kids find it particularly embarrassing to openly discuss these sexual practices.

Once again, progressive coaching can help. This technique will help to reduce any embarrassment you may feel in talking with your kids about this topic, and it can help to combat any embarrassment your kids may experience. After all, this isn't the usual topic of "polite conversation" for them either. Your kids may need help in finding the courage to be open with you about their reactions and curiosities. Remember, the ultimate purpose of all this is to provide your kids with safer sexual alternatives for decreasing their risks of contracting AIDS and other sexually transmitted diseases.

Let's briefly review the use of progressive coaching as a method for "desensitizing" people to activities that feel uncomfortable. As you may recall, by starting with easier, more comfortable activities and gradually progressing to what would otherwise have been distinctly uncomfortable, we replace "pain" with success and growing confidence. Progressive coaching has been applied to all kinds of emotional problems and is one of the most effective and widely used methods in applied psychology. Chapters 3 and 4 have already made extensive use of this technique. Because of the great potential for embarrassment that the topic of alternative sexual practices may hold for you, we'll discuss these methods in some detail in this chapter. Even if you've learned how to use progressive coaching from reading one of the earlier chapters, you may still find some of our suggestions helpful for discussing alternatives to intercourse.

REDUCING YOUR INITIAL EMBARRASSMENT

Applications of progressive coaching can range from the treatment of severe phobias by professional therapists to just reducing milder forms of everyday fears and discomforts. "Desensitizing" people to things that disturb them involves the same principles of progressive coaching that we discuss and apply throughout this book.

If you have a really intense fear of talking about sexual variations or even of talking about sex in general, we hope you'll seek professional help. In fact, we would encourage it, especially if you're serious about AIDS-proofing your kids. On the other hand, if discussing these subjects with your kids causes you just the usual discomforts and anxieties, then you can use progressive coaching to desensitize yourself.

Progressive coaching of yourself, as with progressive coaching of your kids, requires starting at an easy level and progressing through small changes in behavior. Begin with what feels most comfortable and progress slowly toward what would otherwise have felt quite uncomfortable. A decrease in discomfort results with each step along the way. Your goal is to be able to discuss sexual alternatives to intercourse with minimal discomfort and embarrassment.

A simple self-desensitizing procedure involves the following steps and stages:

1. Write down a series of increasingly uncomfortable actions that you will later have to do. These actions should include getting information about sexual variations, informing your kids about them, and all the necessary steps in-between.

2. Once these actions are written down in a list that begins with a relatively easy, minimally uncomfortable action, begin actually doing each action in turn.

3. Progress through the list at a pace slow enough to minimize your discomforts.

4. Return to an easier action if a current one seems too discomforting.

5. Add new actions to try, if necessary, before you try an action that seems too uncomfortable.

Your task here is to become progressively more at ease in considering and communicating sexual alternatives to intercourse. Of course, if you can already do this comfortably, then there's no reason to create this written series, and you should read ahead on how to desensitize your kids.

Once the series of actions are written down in an order of increasing discomfort, you should begin planning how and when to do the first and easiest action.

Let's say that your first action is to go out and buy a magazine or sex manual from the local store. One of the first things you may notice when you attempt this is that you experience a good deal of unexpected discomfort. Browsing through these materials in a store where you're known or where neighbors or friends may stumble upon you is not as easy as you expected. If you experience too much discomfort, don't hesitate to remove yourself from the situation and consider an easier, more comfortable action. Here are some possibilities:

- Go to a store in another neighborhood where you're unlikely to meet people you know.

- Examine a more "mainstream" magazine.

- Start with a more "professional" or "scientific" book.

- Buy the first magazine that looks at all likely and examine it in the privacy of your own home.

- Get books from the library, where you can examine what's available by less conspicuously browsing through the library's card catalog.

Let's say that your next action is to discuss with your spouse the information you're acquiring about sexual variations. We feel that this is a very important action.

Asking your spouse to read the materials with you or to judge their suitability for presentation to your kids could be an embarrassing experience. Some easier, more comfortable actions may have to be taken first. For instance, just being seen by your spouse holding the magazine or book may be easier, if you have first informed your spouse of your intention to purchase one. Or perhaps just mentioning a relatively benign point from it, without naming the source, would be easier still. Later, you can gradually progress to discussing more of what you're reading, perhaps eventually considering variations of your own sexual preferences as well. This might help in reducing the uneasiness with your spouse. Again, you have to be the judge.

By keeping your tasks easy, comfortable, and manageable, you'll progress through your series of actions within days or weeks, depending on your starting point and your experiences along the way, and soon you'll be considering the best way to share your growing knowledge with your kids.

DISCUSSING ALTERNATIVE SEXUAL PRACTICES WITHOUT BLUSHING

Of course, all your knowledge about safer and enjoyable alternatives to sexual intercourse is of little value to your kids if they don't know about them. Their own embarrassments will come to light when you try to inform them.

The same logic of progressive coaching that you may have already applied to your own initial discomforts applies here. You must determine the minimal conditions under which you and your kids can approach this comfortably. The details are particular to your own situation, but we can provide some tips and possible approaches for you to consider.

How to Progressively Coach Alternative Sex

- **Your first step** might involve nothing more than walking into your kids' room with some of your material on alternative sexual practices when your kids aren't around. This may seem silly to you, but if you still shudder at the very idea of approaching your kids on this topic, it is an easy first step, and it should be effective in beginning to reduce some of the discomfort you've been feeling.

- **Your next step** might be to examine some of these materials in your den or living room when your kids are at home. Later you might browse through them, inconspicuously, when your kids are in the room. Identify the minimal conditions that will help you get started and work up from them. Don't be concerned about starting small; success breeds confidence and progress.

- **Next plan some discussions with your spouse.** You and your spouse can prearrange some discussions that will take place in the presence of your kids. These might consist, initially, of only an occasional brief allusion to some aspect of alternative sexual behaviors, such as "You know, you can't get AIDS from hands" or "Fondling is AIDS-proof, right?" or any other remarks that you might find acceptable.

- **Gradually lengthen these discussions with your spouse.** Work in some comments about intercourse being the primary mode for transmission of AIDS and about how people should consider alternative, less risky forms of interpersonal sex. Mention that condoms do fail occasionally. These progressively more explicit interchanges with your spouse could at first be carried out when your kids are just within earshot, but engaged in other activities, perhaps sitting reading in the same room. Later, you could initiate these bits of conversation with your spouse when your kids were in more direct contact with you, such as when you were all sitting around the table together. In this way, you could all begin the process of growing accustomed to having these matters being discussed among you.

- **The perfect opportunity to begin discussing these matters with your kids** will arise when your kids begin to react to any of these remarks or discussions. Any response on their part, short of sheer insolence, should be met with encouragement. Your positive response to their remarks will make them feel much more inclined to share their reactions with you, either then or later.

- **If you have to prod your kids** to get them to start discussing these issues, that's OK too. Be deliberate when you have to, but always be gentle. You might, for starters, ask them and your spouse, too, to look at the materials you now have comfortably at hand that discuss or illustrate sexual techniques not involving intercourse. If you have not found any material that you're prepared to share with them, perhaps just ask them to give some thought to these practices. Later, ask them what they think: Do they feel these ways of enjoying sex are objectionable? Have they ever heard friends or classmates make reference to them? Do they think it's un-manly or unfeminine for people to engage in such prac-tices? Do your kids think that you and your spouse would do these things? Be honest with them!

SOME GENERAL ADVICE

There are a few things to keep in mind as you go through the steps of progressive coaching:

- **Don't expect too much from your kids at first.** Be prepared, if necessary, to present only a single comment or question to them on any one occasion. Be sensitive to their reactions, responding to any sign of excessive dis-comfort by "retreating" to another, nonsexual topic. There will be time enough to try again later. And always be supportive and encouraging to them. Be satisfied with what they can say now. They should be able to say more in the future.

- **There are advantages to having your spouse present for these discussions.** This diffuses the responsibility, and it may make things easier for you. It might also make your kids feel that this is more of a family discus-sion than one centered on them. In fact, trying to maneu-ver the introduction of these topics into ongoing conversations that have set a relaxed tone and keeping your discussions as casual as possible may make them that much less threatening for you and your kids alike.

- **Don't think that humor is out of place.** As long as it doesn't take the form of derogatory or sarcastic remarks, a bit of laughter is a great tension-releaser.

- **Not all these encounters need be perfectly pre-planned.** This is an important point. Take advantage of whatever natural opportunities may come about for you to discuss the topic of sexual alternatives. For example, as we've mentioned earlier in this book, television programs such as sitcoms, soap operas, documentaries, and even news broadcasts are being increasingly explicit about AIDS and sexual practices. They can provide an excellent opportunity to start a conversation with your kids. Use these situations as a natural springboard for discussion. You should keep your eye on reviews of current films or videos and previews of television shows so as to identify any that may contain scenes or topics for you to consider with your kids. Using the entertainment media to your advantage can be a welcome relief from the exploitation we all sometimes feel.

- **Don't forget reward.** Meaningful and tangible benefits, promised in return for participation in minimal discussions, may be all your kids need to get started talking. A willingness to get more involved in these issues with you, even if it is based on the selfish pursuit of tangible rewards, may grow into a genuine commitment. Once they begin to consider ways of protecting their lives without having to give up their desires for sexual enjoyment, their learning becomes its own reward.

The goal that you are approaching, ever so slowly but comfortably for all of you, is being able to talk about sexual matters as comfortably as you might talk about favorite foods, redecorating your rooms, neutering your pet, or other such family matters. Such sexual activities as mutual masturbation, oral sex, nonorgasmic sexual play, and the use of vibrators should become family topics of discussion, along with consideration of the AIDS-related risks involved.

USE OF ROLE-PLAYS

In Chapter 4, we presented a number of role-plays to help get your kids to insist on the use of a condom with a partner reluctant to do so. If your kids are to opt for sexual alternatives to intercourse, they may run into the same problem. The fact that they are knowledgeable, possibly even experts, in these sexual variations may be enough to convince their partners that full satisfaction can be achieved without intercourse. But verbal arguments might be needed, too. And practice, under conditions designed to be as realistic as possible, may be needed to learn how to refuse to have intercourse as a means of sexual expression. We therefore suggest that you consider using role-plays similar to those in Chapter 4. How elaborate these are to be is up to you and your kids to work out. Use a style of speech that is comfortable and reasonable for your kids. Even a statement as simple as "I've decided that if I'm going to feel safe, I'm just not going to have intercourse" might be enough to work on. Progressive coaching and realistic practice with statements such as this can help your kids acquire some of the certainty and decisiveness they need to convince a partner.

We'll provide you with two examples of role-plays. Remember to treat these only as starting points for your own versions that you develop and change with your kids. And don't forget to give your kids lots of praise, approval, and material rewards, if necessary, for each of their repeated attempts, no matter how clumsy they may sometimes be.

Boy Resisting Alternatives to Intercourse

BOY: You've got to let me come inside you.

GIRL: I told you, I'll help you come, and I promise you'll enjoy it — you'll see.

BOY: It isn't natural. I'll even use a condom. I thought we loved each other.

GIRL: We do love each other. That doesn't mean we shouldn't be careful.

BOY: I told you I haven't slept with anyone except you, so you don't have to worry about AIDS. Don't you trust me?

GIRL: (**Note:** *There's no way to refute this argument, so she shouldn't try.*) It makes me feel safest to avoid intercourse, and that's the decision I've made for myself. If you respect my feelings, you'll accept this, instead of looking for reasons to change my mind. I don't intend to change my mind, no matter what you say.

BOY: We've talked about getting married some day. Aren't we going to make love when we are married?

GIRL: When we get married, we'll do it. (*She fondles his penis.*) I promise you'll enjoy what I'm going to do. Let's find out what you like . . . .

Girl Resisting Alternatives to Intercourse

GIRL: I told you, I don't like it unless you're inside me. Just let me put this condom on you . . . . (*She prepares to apply condom.*)

BOY: (*Stands up to avoid condom and to avoid caresses that may get him excited enough to lose his resolve.*) I want you to like it, and I want to, too, and I'm not doing this to be mean. I've made a decision that the only way I can stop worrying about AIDS is if I avoid any way that isn't one hundred percent safe.

GIRL: You think I'm infected, don't you?

BOY: Of course not. I don't think that. It's got nothing to do with whether or not you're infected. I'm just saying that this is the only way I won't worry. I'm asking you to respect my decision because it feels right for me.

GIRL: And what am I supposed to do when I don't like it?

BOY: (*Ignoring extreme statements and getting down to it.*) I like this (*snuggling close and comforting*) and you do too . . . .

These scripts may not be exactly what your kids might say; they may not even come close. That's why it's important that you work with them to develop scripts that they are comfortable with and then practice (reward), practice (reward), and practice!

IF YOU CAN'T QUITE PULL IT OFF

We recognize that some of you will not openly discuss alternative sexual practices with your kids, either because you're unable to or because you've chosen not to. Nevertheless, you'll want at least to get information about these sexual variations into your kids' hands.

The printed materials that you acquire, or some selection of them, can be given outright to your kids with little or no explanation. Chances are that they'll accept them and read them without coaxing from you. Of course, there's no reason why you can't just leave publications around in conspicuous places to be looked at or taken away by your kids. Be careful, though; don't make "cute" or teasing comments about how the materials have disappeared. This can serve only to embarrass your kids and make them even more reluctant to discuss sexual alternatives with you.

It should not be a cause for panic if you're not able to discuss these matters openly with your kids at this time. Sharing the materials you have acquired in a noninteractive way may become a springboard for eventual talking. Try it and see.

In any case, take some action. Don't let your fear cause you to postpone addressing this with your kids. Although your kids will likely be exposed to various printed and graphic materials on the streets, you can't be assured of this. Nor can you be assured that you would approve of what they might come across on their own. If your kids are to find out about appropriate sexual alternatives to intercourse, it's best for them to find this out from you, whether you arrange it in an interactive way or not. We remind you once again, however, that a full appreciation and wholesome attitude toward alternatives to intercourse is best achieved through your guidance.

Keep in mind that kids who can develop nonintercourse ways of enjoying sex and satisfying their partners are more AIDS-safe than before. It's a changed world, and we can't ignore it!

6

Help the Schools: They Desperately Need It

We appreciate that this problem of safeguarding our kids from AIDS is not an easy problem to think about, let alone to act upon.

Not all of you will do and say all that we have suggested. Some of you will find it impossible to do much of anything we have suggested. If you've found the exercises and topics we've outlined so far to be too much for you, there's a responsible "way out." You can ensure that your kids receive and profit from other educational opportunities. Get involved in your local school's efforts to make kids more AIDS-safe. And if even this is more than you're able to do, perhaps your spouse or a close and trusted friend might, at your suggestion, take on the responsibility of AIDS-proofing, with or without your participation.

Getting closely involved with your kids' school is also good advice for those of you who are able to do a lot of what we've advocated so far. The efforts being made by your local school can be a valuable supplement to your family's efforts.

To help you, we've listed some organizations at the end of Chapter 10 that will assist schools in educating kids on the issues of AIDS. Take on the task of using the phone numbers we've provided so that you can call and evaluate what these organizations can do for you and your kids' school. This is important, especially if your local school is not doing much in the way of AIDS-proofing. Make one phone call today and another tomorrow on behalf of your school, on behalf of your kids. You don't need the school's permission to make these calls. You don't need an approval from teachers. You need only an appreciation for the risks your kids face. Try to get an assurance from these organizations that they will help your kids' school. Start today.

Many teachers are currently developing or delivering curriculum to help our kids understand and cope with the risks of AIDS. These teachers are, at a minimum, providing information on AIDS and, if possible within accepted community standards, on the practice of safer sex and/or abstinence.

We could simply urge you to get involved with your school's efforts, but we believe that's inadequate. Instead, as we've done throughout this book, we're giving you actual steps you should take to make your involvement effective. Here are your goals:

- Identify teachers who are addressing the AIDS issue.

- Give the teachers very specific and needed support.

- Help your kids fully participate in the classroom so as to optimize their education on AIDS.

- Become a resource for both your kids and the teachers.

- Help create a parent/community environment that will further your kids' chances at survival.

IDENTIFY THE TEACHERS

One or more of the teachers in your kids' school are likely to be involved with a so-called "sex-education" or "family-life" course. Find the teachers who are instructing the course or who hope to instruct it. In our experience, it is best to deal directly with teachers. School boards and administrators are considerably more conservative and cautious and will be of limited help to you. Teachers who have agreed or volunteered to teach sex-related topics are usually highly motivated on the issue of AIDS education. These are the teachers to contact and work with.

HOW TO GIVE SUPPORT

In many cases, teachers are uncertain as to how parents will react to their teaching about AIDS. The teachers' uncertainties, along with the usually more timid attitudes of their administrators and school board, leave them in a vulnerable position. They'll need you to be clear, explicit, and obvious in your support of them.

We urge you to express your concerns to teachers in concrete ways. This means more than just expressing that AIDS education is necessary. It will be all too easy for you to fall into simple, head-nodding agreements with the teachers without really letting them know that you're fully in support of frank and forthright teaching. You must show them that you want your kids to get the best instruction with as few compromises as possible.

Your support of the teachers can be helped by specifying the types of AIDS-proofing skills outlined so far in this book. It might be useful to loan the teachers a copy of this book, if they don't already have one. This could help to make explicit what you may find too embarrassing to say.

By being explicit as to exactly what skills you want your kids to learn, you'll be doing the teachers a favor in their dealings with administrators. The teachers are likely under administrative pressure to keep their teachings vague and thus "harmless" and noncontroversial. Your expectations, being different, will lend courage and conviction to the teachers in their proposals to colleagues and administrators.

By being explicit as to what skills you want your kids to learn, you'll be doing your kids a favor too. You'll be helping to ensure that they'll have a course taught to them which deals with more than just their awareness, attitudes, and feelings. This is not to say that awareness, attitudes, and feelings aren't important, but it's the skills they learn that could save their lives. These can be the skills of safer sex or the skills involved in abstaining from interpersonal sex.

HOW TO PREPARE YOUR KIDS
FOR CLASSROOM PARTICIPATION

Kids are usually reluctant to speak up in class or to ask questions, even under the best of circumstances. They're particularly unlikely to do so when the topics are as potentially embarrassing and controversial as the issues surrounding AIDS. Having your kids simply be present in a classroom does little to ensure that they'll learn anything.

Whatever the nature of the course that is taught to your kids, they will get a better experience by being active and co-operative participants. And teachers can be more straightforward in their presentation of sensitive issues if they see that one or more students are eager to learn. Try to put yourself in the teachers' position. They are facing a large number of kids who will giggle, snicker, wince, fidget, or just blankly stare when sex or sex-related issues are mentioned. These are hardly the conditions under which to expect an already professionally vulnerable and perhaps personally uneasy teacher to teach.

Just how receptive will your kids be to learning about AIDS protection in the school classroom? The answer to this is, in part, up to you.

At one extreme, by having read this book and successfully done what was recommended, you'll be giving the teachers a well-informed kid who is relatively at ease with the topic. This can't help but enrich the classroom experience. Your kid, by breaking the ice, will be encouraging other kids in the class to speak up as well. With more kids talking, and thus more viewpoints aired, issues may arise that could supplement the teacher's materials. In fact, issues may arise that might never have arisen in your own discussions with your kids. This could be an unforeseen benefit of your kids' participation with their peers at school.

At the other extreme, you may be so very uncomfortable with this entire issue of AIDS and sex that you have done little with your kids on the topics raised in this book. Your kids may likely share this discomfort and, in addition, they will not have received the possible instructional benefits of this book. They may be rather unprepared, uncomfortable, and unreceptive to their teacher's instruction.

In either case, you will want your kids to participate fully in class so they acquire all the skills and information presented.

Although much of your kids' participation in class will be under the control of their teachers, two types of participation can be enhanced by you. One type involves your kids asking questions for clarification, such as, "You say it's safer, but what exactly is oral sex?" Will your kids be likely to ask a question like this, or will they just be thinking it? The other type involves your kids suggesting elaborations or entire topics that are not being covered, such as, "There's other ways of having fun, you know, than just doing that intercourse stuff."

Making the instruction complete and worthwhile is more than just the teacher's responsibility, especially when the teacher may be somewhat embarrassed, timid, vulnerable, or intimidated by uncooperative parents or colleagues.

Your kids' questioning and opening up more avenues of discussion may not come easy to them, but it can be made less "painful" by your coordinated efforts with the teacher.

It is doubtful that your kids need any progressive coaching on the mechanics of how to ask a question or how to suggest a possible topic for discussion. They likely do know how, at least well enough to be understood. Their problem will likely be one of sufficient motivation. They'll have to have strong incentives to overcome the uneasiness or embarrassment of speaking up in class on the topic of sex.

Your job, then, with the help of the teacher, will be to provide for their motivation. You'll have to give them sufficient incentive to begin and perhaps to continue to speak up.

We have suggested elsewhere in this book that you should not be reluctant to make contracts with your kids. In this case, you must consider offering them special privileges or material incentives in return for their active participation in class. The participation can be confirmed by the teacher. Again, don't think of this as bribery, which is the use of incentives for purposes of exploitation. It is clearly in your kids' own best interest to ask questions and to help steer or prod the teacher into specifying the actual AIDS-proofing skills that must be learned.

With progressive coaching in mind, the participation of your kids should at first be minimal, with the demands increasing gradually over time. Classroom questions from your kids can initially be brief, simple, benign, and even written privately to the teacher, rather than spoken in class, such as, "Can you speak a little louder?"

Your kids' suggestions for topics can likewise be initially comfortable and noncontroversial, such as, "Will you please talk about whether AIDS can be cured." But a close coordination with the teacher will be necessary to arrange for this and to arrange for the progressive increase in your kids' degree of participation. You will need daily confirmation from the teacher as to your kids' successes so that the incentives you are holding can be validly awarded: "Hey, good going. Your teacher said you got in a question today. Here's the TV guide; it's your choice tonight."

Getting involved with the school in this manner may let you off the hook from discussing sex with your kids. But you'll need an ongoing commitment and involvement with their teachers, because they'll be the ones engaging in the potentially embarrassing discussions. Anything less than this will not permit you to use your incentives. And, as we've pointed out, without incentives, your kids may not be effectively participating in the class. Don't leave their participation to chance.

HOW TO BE A RESOURCE TO YOUR KIDS AND THEIR TEACHERS

If your kids' teachers are truly teaching the skills involved in AIDS prevention, then don't be shocked if your kids need to take a condom to class. In fact, if the teachers are not instructing the kids on the use of condoms, you'll want your kids to ask for this, thereby giving the teacher some courage and support to do so. In either case, you may have to provide the condoms or, better yet, under the teachers' instructions, give your kids the money to buy them. (See Chapter 4 for a discussion of this issue.)

Your kids' teachers may also need examples of magazines or manuals that cover topics relevant to safer sex. (See Chapter 5 for a discussion of this issue.) Be prepared and willing to help. Your willingness to help will be taken as a sign of your support. Keep yourself reminded of their professional vulnerability and personal discomfort about the subject of AIDS. They need your help.

Some teachers give homework assignments to their students on sex- and AIDS-related topics. For example, questionnaires about family expectations regarding sexual practices are not uncommon. Be prepared to be an honest and open resource for your kids. Any sense of embarrassment from you at times like this could be reflected in your kids' own subsequent shyness in class.

Some teachers may want their students to get together and "rap" on the topics raised in class. Be prepared to allow your kids the time to meet with their friends, and provide them the space to meet in, if necessary.

Be prepared to set aside your own comforts and values for the sake of your child's education. Be willing to provide whatever your kids or their teachers may need from you. You've given the schools a tough task, made tougher by the fact that they, unlike you, are a publicly accountable institution answerable to other parents.

GATHER LIKE-MINDED
PARENTS FOR SUPPORT

Make no mistake about it, there are parents who would never consider addressing the issue of AIDS prevention with their kids. Some of these same parents will object to classroom consideration of this topic, too.

This places the schools in a particularly awkward position, and it's worth repeating that it also places concerned teachers in a very vulnerable position. The school administrators and the teachers need all the public support they can get if they are to educate kids on the topic of AIDS-safe habits.

Here are some ideas of ways in which you can give your school and teachers your individual support:

- If you are skilled at writing, submit some letters to the editor of your local newspaper. This will help to get the issues out in public view.

- Contact your local community cable television studio. Offer them a panel composed of healthcare and educational professionals and parents to discuss the issues involved in AIDS-proofing kids. Use this book and/or other publications as a springboard for discussion. You can avoid, if necessary, the possible embarrassment of a public appearance by being just the organizer of this event. There are many professionals who are trained to take the heat of public debate and who have the experience to be on the front lines. These or similar events provide the community atmosphere in which our schools can begin to act.

- If you are skilled at talking and letting your beliefs be known, drop by the staff room at your school to have coffee and talk with individual teachers. A few such "drop-ins" will quickly identify those teachers who are in sympathy with your concerns, but take the first few coffee breaks with them on less controversial issues. Remember progressive coaching. Eventually you can show your support for their sympathy on the AIDS issue and try to work this sympathy into action.

- Try to gain support for your school from the local parent/teachers' association. Parents are the adults in the community to whom the teachers are most answerable and from whom the teachers are most in need of support. But enlist support with the same care as we've asked you to take in dealing with all problems of coaching behavior. Use progressive coaching. Thus, don't go to an association meeting and demand support right off the mark for full-scale AIDS-prevention courses. Rather, gradually raise your concerns in nonthreatening, informal ways, initially voicing your concerns individually only to seemingly like-minded parents. Use only noncontroversial language at first, such as "AIDS prevention" rather than "safer sex" and "AIDS protection" rather than "use of condoms." If there are no sex-education courses currently operating in your school, consider asking for minimal inclusion of AIDS-awareness in already existing courses in the curriculum. In our experience there are likely one or more teachers who have been waiting for such an expression of support to act. Your initial cautiousness and progressively greater demands will likely keep a number of parents with you with you and will avoid alienating any timid or vulnerable teaching staff.

With growing support from other parents, jointly you can slowly increase your demands. Your goal should be to ask for and receive the teaching of actual skills to your kids, such as the skills presented in this book. In fact, for some of you, this may be your kids' only chance to learn these skills before they have to be used and used effectively.

Along the way, however, you may find yourself falling into a trap of premature comfort and ease. It is often all too easy for us to be satisfied with mutual promises to one another to help the kids toward "AIDS-awareness," "appropriate attitudes toward sex," and "getting in touch with feelings." These are very popular phrases right now. Too often, however, these wonderfully sounding phrases are a substitute for getting down to the real task of teaching specific skills. These ideas may strike a sympathetic chord, but it's the learning of actual skills for safer sex or abstinence that will prevent the suffering and deaths we can otherwise expect.

PART III

Teaching Alternatives to
Interpersonal Sex

7

"No Sex Please": The Option of Abstinence

Some of you may be thinking that we've been missing the boat, that the only sure way to avoid AIDS is simply to abstain from interpersonal sex completely. You may have special reasons for feeling this way. Your kids may be at high risk because of the nature of their neighborhood or friends, or your moral code may preclude your kids from having sex under their present circumstances. Whatever your reasons, you may want your kids to defer their sexual activities until their situation is safer and/or more appropriate.

ABSTINENCE OR SAFER SEX — WHICH ONE?

It is not for us to make value judgments on whether it is best for you to teach safer sex or abstinence from interpersonal sex. Such a decision is yours to make, because you are the only one informed enough about your family situation. There are, however, some hard, practical issues that must be considered. Most important, it is unrealistic to depend on just

103

prohibiting your kids from having sex. No matter how obedient and well-meaning they may be, they are nonetheless creatures of biology. Given the right circumstances, passion may override even the best of intentions. And the "right circumstances" might be something as ordinary and innocent as time alone with the one they're currently in love with.

One way to deal with the possibility that your kids may "accidently stumble" into sex is to make sure they are adequately prepared. This means coaching them in the protective methods discussed in earlier chapters. This is our personal recommendation. You may reject this approach, perhaps through concern that such coaching might increase the likelihood of your kids having sex. We can't guarantee you otherwise. So we urge you to give this issue some serious deliberation, perhaps with your family as a whole, before making your decision.

In discussing these issues with your kids, however, be prepared for unrealistic promises. Kids can easily promise abstinence with either the best of intentions or as a means of ending the discussion about sex that you're insisting on having with them. Words have an unhappy habit of not predicting actions. Don't ever end the topic of AIDS-proofing with them on just the basis of promises. Actions do indeed speak louder than words, and we will continue to advise you to coach actions, even on this topic of abstinence.

IF YOU STILL CHOOSE ABSTINENCE

Your only alternative, if you reject instruction in safer sex, is to make sure that your kids do not have the opportunity to engage in sex. This means that any contact they have with other kids must either be under direct supervision of a responsible adult or must occur in public settings where sex would be extremely unlikely or difficult. A more extreme strategy would be to try to get your kids to spend more time by themselves.

Don't misunderstand us. We are not suggesting that any time kids get together without adult scrutiny they'll immediately have sex. That is nonsense. But if you've decided on abstinence from interpersonal sex as the means for AIDS-proofing your kids, then you have little choice. You've got to try to keep those occasions where a sexual encounter is possible to a minimum. Of course, restricting the nature or extent of your kids' social activities may involve some cost for them. This cost is their reduced opportunities to learn social skills and to experience nonthreatening and important forms of intimacy with other kids. This, too, should be a factor in your decision.

FIND ENJOYABLE, SEX-FREE ALTERNATIVES FOR YOUR KIDS

This chapter covers how to minimize the risk that your kids will engage in interpersonal sex by maximizing their participation and enjoyment in activities that are sex-free. Behavioral scientists have repeatedly found that threats, warnings, and punishments usually work only while kids are within reach. You'll be unlikely to succeed at preventing interpersonal sex using these methods, because your kids are not always in reach. You do have a reasonable likelihood of succeeding if you try to develop enjoyable alternatives for your kids instead.

Your task, whatever leisure activities you choose to encourage, is to do everything in your power to ensure that:

• Alternative activities provide no opportunities for sex

- Your kids get thoroughly caught up in enjoying these sex-free activities.

You don't have a prayer of stopping kids from the pleasures of intimate contact unless you've got some very pleasurable alternatives for them. Succeeding in your goal may require a considerable sacrifice of time from you, both for your planning and for your subsequent involvement. One place to start in your search for enjoyable, nonsexual activities is to note how your kids choose to spend their time now:

- Are they continually out on the playing field? Soccer and sex are difficult to do at the same time, as is the case with most other group sports.

- Do they love to swim? Sex in a public swimming pool is unlikely.

- Do they read, watch television, or listen to records a lot? Alone-time may allow solo sexual activity, but it can't involve interpersonal sex.

- Do they play a musical instrument? Private or group music lessons and group music performances do not provide opportunities for sex.

These or similar activities that qualify as being AIDS-safe should provide a natural starting point for you — people usually choose to do things they enjoy. The following sections provide some more ideas, with special considerations and suggestions for promoting your kids' participation in AIDS-safe leisure activities.

ACTIVITIES WITH OTHER KIDS

There are many ways for your kids to have fun with other kids while minimizing their risk of sexual encounters. The key idea is that one usually can't have sex while in public view, especially if an adult is present, so an important characteristic of AIDS-safe activities is that they occur in public.

Community Groups

Most communities offer a variety of kid-oriented social or team-sports activities and clubs, either through schools, churches, recreational centers, or other organizations. Kids who are busy in well-supervised, organized groups are generally safe from sexual encounters. Your main problem here is one of determining whether your kids will find enough enjoyment in these activities to maintain their attendance. Use these hints to decide if you have chosen activities that best fit your child's needs and desires.

- **Watch your kids!** Note their laughter, smiles, good cheer, and general demeanor. Are they having fun? Don't count on other parents to let you know. They may have gone to great lengths to get their own kids involved and could be reluctant to admit to any problems. Especially don't count on the judgments of your kid's enjoyment by adult chaperons, coaches, or organizers — they often have a vested interest in painting a rosy picture.

- **Go and see for yourself,** in an unobtrusive way to avoid your kids' complaining about your presence. They're your kids and you're usually the best person to judge their feelings. If possible, get involved as a cosupervisor or adult chaperon so that you can have some personal control over the particular activities your kids get involved in. This can ensure that outings, sports games, socials, dances, and the like are geared toward kids not pairing off in isolating ways that might encourage sexual encounters. Don't forget, you may be the only adult there who is seeking AIDS-safe, enjoyable social interactions. So get active!

Getting Your Kids to Join

You may encounter resistance from your kids to the notion of joining a community group. They may be shy about joining new group activities or prefer to just "hang out" with their friends. But if you have reason to believe that they would enjoy certain group activities in spite of their objections, then you'll have to take some steps to get them involved.

Once you've identified some potentially enjoyable group activities for your kids, how do you get them to participate?

- **Provide wheels.** One initial step you must take is to make it easy for them to participate. Drive them to and from the activity if you have to, especially the first time.

- **Provide a buddy.** See if you can get one or more of their friends to join with them. If having friends with them is still not enough to get your kids to participate, then be prepared to take advantage of your greater financial clout.

- **Provide "goodies."** Kids usually don't have the resources to pay for all the things they'd like to do or buy. You do — at least more than they do. Negotiate a deal with them. If they attend two or more sessions of a group activity, you agree to give them a contribution toward that special purchase they've been saving for, or a couple of free CDs, or a raise in their allowance for as long as they attend. Your options are unlimited, so be creative.

The reward must depend on your kids abiding by the conditions you've both agree upon. As we've said before, this kind of behavioral contracting is a common feature of many currently popular parenting techniques. But to make negotiations work you've got to have darn good "goodies" on your side of the table. Remember that you're competing against the highly rewarding activity of "just hanging out"!

Although material rewards for starting AIDS-safe activities are often the best, don't forget that other potential resource — your approval. This will, of course, vary in effectiveness from family to family, as some parents have better rapport and influence with their kids than others. Depending on your circumstances, a sincere request coupled with an honest explanation of your concern might work. This might be all it takes for your kids to agree to become involved in group and other AIDS-safe social activities.

Homemade Groups

If community-based groups or team sports activities are not possible or promise little enjoyment for your kids, then "Super-Parent" may have to come to the rescue. Organize your own fully supervised get-togethers. These might include:

- Dance parties
- Video or game nights
- Group outings to local, highly prized attractions

- Neighborhood sports matches, such as basketball, baseball, or volleyball.

Any activity will do as long as it allows your kids to get together socially and safely with other kids. The key is your active participation, with a few like-minded parents, in the planning of the activity and in the event itself. You may run the risk of being labelled an overcontrolling or nontrusting parent, but a couple of successful social events loaded with pizza can often overcome all such objections.

Getting your kids to agree to any of these homemade activities or to the particular conditions you attach to them will require that they be fairly receptive to your suggestions. Many parents, particularly those with older teenagers, may encounter some difficulties with this. Once again some monetary investment may help. You should be willing and eager to pay for the VCR and videos, pizza for the gang after the volleyball game, or for some of the sports equipment your kids and their friends want, perhaps with some help from other like-minded parents as well.

These kinds of incentives—food and money—can make your kids and their friends more cooperative. Of course, organizing and participating in these activities is going to mean a large investment of your time and resources. You may have to seriously shift your personal priorities, perhaps more so than you're accustomed to in parenting. We think the payoff will be worth it and will take you a long way toward AIDS-proofing your kids.

A Note of Caution

You may feel that same-sex activities are completely safe. The evidence, however, is that sexual contact among kids of the same sex is not at all uncommon. It may occur at a relatively young age and often has little or nothing to do with "natural" homosexual or heterosexual inclinations. Same-sex, intimate contact may vary from one community to the next, but the mere possibility just reinforces the basic imperative we have been stressing here: social activities must be either within public view or under adult supervision to be maximally risk-free from AIDS.

ACTIVITIES FOR THE INDIVIDUAL KID

Many leisure activities, because they are taught and can be carried out on an individual basis, are basically incompatible with sexual encounters.

Community-based Activities

One set of activities for kids that is incompatible with sexual encounters is instructor-led lessons in recreational and artistic skills. In the learning of many such skills, social interactions between kids are relatively minimal and are also under the observation of a teacher. Some examples include:

- Lessons in music, art, writing, and other individual pursuits
- Lessons or coaching in individually competitive sports such as archery, golf, gymnastics, skating, and swimming
- Lessons in other activities from cooking or weaving to electronics and computers.

Anything that provides an opportunity for kids to gain personal and useful skills while also enjoying themselves can be considered. The key is that gaining expertise must not be done at the expense of enjoyment. You are developing these opportunities for your kids as a pleasurable alternative to one of nature's most pleasurable experiences — interpersonal intimacy and sex. You've got to do everything you can to ensure that these alternative activities will be enjoyable. Some things you can do to make these activities more enjoyable for your kids are:

- **Provide wheels.** Make it easy for your kids by driving them to and from their lessons.

- **Root for them.** Be uncritical of their efforts. Be unequivocal in your praise, no matter how slow or small their progress may seem. Every hour here is an AIDS-safe hour.

- **Leave your ego behind.** You must set aside your personal hopes for their excellence and artistic accomplishment. It is unlikely that these activities will become their lifetime careers. Work for their satisfaction. No strings of parental ego should be attached or you may begin criticizing or pushing too hard.

Remember, you are trying to maximize the chances of their continued participation in behaviors that are incompatible with having sex.

Home-based Activities

Many leisure activities are solitary in nature and thus go a long way toward AIDS-proofing your kids. Admittedly, if used too heavily, these solitary activities do not help your kids acquire valuable social skills. We feel that social skills are extremely important, but you may have well-founded AIDS worries that warrant temporarily isolating your kids. Solitary activities can provide meaningful enjoyment as well as the opportunity to develop worthwhile personal skills and interests.

Many hobbies, for example, require the participation of only one person:

- Amateur astronomy, which is done at night when others may be out socializing and engaging in sexual behavior
- Stamp and coin collecting
- Woodworking in a home workshop
- Photography and printing in a bathroom/darkroom
- Quilting, sewing, clothes making
- Gardening
- Reading
- That old antisocial standby, television

Your local library or crafts store will be able to suggest many other possibilities.

Once again, the key to getting your kids to engage in solitary activities is to make their participation as pleasurable as you can. This will take some time and effort on your part, particularly for those activities demanding technical abilities. Don't just go out and buy your kids the newest telescope, complete with the latest star charts and flashy posters of the universe. Instead, spend a lot of hours with them, showing interest in their new hobby. You need to be guiding, praising, and generally sharing your kids' experience in the beginning if you want them to stick with it. This is true for almost any solitary activity that you wish to see developed — a lot of early success and gratification has to take place. Remember the technique for progressive coaching: help them to enjoy their initial efforts. Don't count on your kids to succeed right off the mark, although it may sometimes happen. Their continued involvement in these "safe" activities is too important to leave to luck.

Television as a Temporary, Home-based Activity

Socially isolated activities, such as being a "couch potato" in front of the television, usually do not require much adult support. Television seems to have its own built-in, if socially questionable, rewards. But even here, some usual parental habits can get in the way. Be aware that any time you attempt to censor or significantly change your kids' viewing habits you run the risk of diluting the reward value of the television. We certainly aren't advocating that you set no limits at all, but we must caution you that some of your values may have to be compromised. If, in your particular circumstances, the risk of AIDS warrants temporarily keeping your kids at home more and having them watch television, then some changes may have to be made. Remember that you want to make watching television an enjoyable alternative to being out at night, perhaps parked at the local "not-so-AIDS-safe" beach or park.

Letting your kids watch marginal or junky television is not the only option you have in getting them more interested in this safe, home-based activity. There are also many quality programs that your kids might enjoy watching. Well-produced dramas or documentaries need not be inherently dry and boring. In our experience, many kids have just never adequately sampled quality television. In such cases, you only need to provide a valued incentive to get them to try out a good program. A valued incentive might be nothing more than relief from clearing the dinner table that night. Quality programs can be found on public television and on some cable channels. Pick carefully, at first, so you provide a program content that is likely to match your kids' current tastes. And don't forget the progressive coaching!

Most importantly, join your kids for television viewing. Make it a family time with good humor and popcorn. Your participation can be an effective reward, especially if they have only limited access to you due to your work or other personal commitments. If your circumstances temporarily warrant home confinement as an AIDS-safe alternative, a kid at home watching television with you is a kid who is temporarily safe from AIDS.

STRATEGIES NEEDING LESS OF YOUR TIME

Before leaving the topic of solitary activities, we would like to mention some less intrusive steps than we've considered. Be warned, however, that these options may also be less effective because they involve less of your direct participation. Consider providing your kids with:

- Their own book-club membership to encourage more reading
- Their own television set to encourage more staying at home
- More of any hobby materials they might need
- Their own telephone line for socializing in "safety."

Once again, we don't like the idea of kids' losing important opportunities to be together. But if your circumstances really demand a more socially restrictive environment, then it's got to be set up effectively, and this may mean temporarily compromising other parenting concerns until your kids' situation is safer.

ABSTINENCE MEANS SAYING "NO" TO SEX

We have already cautioned that in spite of your careful efforts your kids may still find themselves in a situation where someone proposes having sex with them. They may need some coaching in refusing such advances. The role-play approach that we recommended earlier in this book is useful here as well. You want your kids not only to prepare some ways of politely and sensitively declining sexual proposi-tions, but of doing so in a way that is least likely to prompt an argument or an insult or to result in coercion. They must learn and rehearse how to do this — these skills are not handed out at birth.

- Ask your kids if they or their friends have experienced sexual advances. If needed, progressively coach them in their ability to talk with you about this.

- Start with easy topics and slowly work up to the more intimate conversations. What form did these sexual ad-vances take? What type of response seemed most effec-tive? Did they have any particular problems?

- Use the information to prepare some scripts to practice with.

The following example, similar to the one provided in Chapter 4, might serve as a starting point. It depicts a girl re-fusing the advances of a boy. With minor changes, it could just as readily be used for a boy refusing the advances of a girl. This is just one example, though, and any scripts that you develop should be done together with your kids in their own words and style. Be careful — don't make fun of their ways of expression, and be tolerant of their making fun of you.

Girl Saying No to Sex

BOY: You've really got me excited. I want to make love to you.

GIRL: I like you too, _____, a lot. But because of the AIDS scare, my parents and I have agreed that I'm not going to have sex yet — no matter how much I might want to.

BOY: But I thought you liked me.

GIRL: I *do* like you. But I've made a commitment to myself and to my parents. I hope you'll respect that.

BOY: But if you do like me, and if you want to have sex with me, then I don't see why we can't. I'll use a condom, and I'll be very careful, so there's really no risk at all.

GIRL: Please, _____. I know how you feel, and I don't blame you, but this is a decision that everyone has to make for themselves. I've made my decision, and if you care about me, you won't try to talk me out of it. I really feel strongly about that.

A script like this, or one more suited to your special circumstances and to the language of your kids, is only a beginning. It would be wise for you and your kids to develop the actual pleas and refusals that could be encountered under more stubborn circumstances. Consider scenarios in which verbal refusals are no longer sufficient. How can one partner physically leave an interaction in safety? Rehearse and practice it. Can you count on your kid being able to approach adults or other kids for help? You can't count on your kids to seek help from other sources unless the actions required are actually rehearsed and practiced.

It takes practice to create the courage to get out of a car stopped at an intersection. It takes practice to create the courage to approach strangers, police cars, or unfamiliar homes on an unfamiliar street to seek help. Yet these are all possible realities in the course of refusing sex. These corrective actions must be practiced. Words of assurance from your kids that they're capable must not be accepted as sufficient. The stakes are too high!

Progressive coaching, the use of role-plays, and the use of effective incentives and rewards, as we've outlined throughout this book, will allow you to set up and carry out simulations of these various scenarios. Words alone are not a good enough substitute for real-life practice. Do it!

8

Masturbation: You Can't Get AIDS from Yourself

The topic of alternatives to interpersonal sex would not be complete without consideration of the alternative sexual outlet provided by masturbation.

This topic is rather difficult to introduce, as we recognize that many parents feel uneasy about their kids engaging in masturbation. We can only say, as we've said before, that the value judgments are yours to make. All we can do is to provide potentially useful suggestions. Masturbation is a viable and AIDS-proof alternative to interpersonal sex. Its widespread practice among both kids and adults is a fact. It would be naive to believe otherwise.

WHY YOUR KIDS NEED YOUR ADVICE

You'll be correct in assuming that your kids will require little encouragement to engage in this AIDS-proof alternative. The pleasure of masturbation provides its own encouragement. Nonetheless, there are two areas in which your input is needed:

- **Social taboos.** Your kids have likely encountered social taboos against masturbation. You should consider countering these influences if you're intent on your kids having an AIDS-proof, noninterpersonal sexual outlet.

- **They don't know how.** Your kids may not know exactly how to get sufficient enjoyment from masturbation. You should consider providing them with valid information on this topic. The techniques for maximizing pleasure in masturbation are likely learned over the years, well into adulthood. Kids, especially girls, may fail to develop a full enjoyment of masturbation during the time in which they could most use it as an AIDS-proof, noninterpersonal sexual outlet.

INFORMING YOUR KIDS

You'll be able to find material on masturbation techniques, as well as on sexuality in general, in bookstores, libraries, and through mail order. You can use the list of Further Readings at the end of Chapter 10 and contact some of the groups listed in the back of the book to get more information. Some are prepared specifically for kids and some are oriented more specifically to female sexuality, young and old.

If discussing this topic with your kids makes you too uncomfortable, you can simply provide these materials for them to read on their own. If your kids feel guilt or concern about masturbation, presenting them with publications of this kind with your active endorsement should help dispel their fears.

You may rightly feel the need to do more than just pass on information to your kids. Cultural or social taboos can be difficult to overcome. You may also wish to overcome the influences of your kids' friends, if you feel their attitudes are having a negative effect on your kids' desire to try masturbation. You may further want to share your own knowledge and attitudes about masturbation with your kids. A more active role for you might entail carefully examining published materials before making them available to your kids. You could then provide the most useful information in the form of photocopies of selected parts or pages. More intimate discussions with your kids, however, will have a far greater impact on their attitudes and understanding of masturbation.

For more in-depth discussions with your kids, you may again employ progressive coaching as outlined in previous chapters:

- First, read some written material on the subject of masturbation while in view of your kids.

- Next, have printed materials available around the house for your kids to browse through. This may even encourage them to initiate discussions with you.

- Proceed to a few mutually agreed-upon remarks to your spouse, in proximity to your kids: "You know, this AIDS issue really leaves kids with no other option than masturbation." "Did you read the title of that chapter, 'Masturbation: You Can't Get AIDS from Yourself'?" The content of these remarks must be mutually agreed upon with your spouse so that your words don't come out of nowhere, producing clumsy reactions. You must customize the content to your situation, but the principle is clear: make the content as comfortable as you can for yourselves and your kids.

- Finally, direct discussions with your kids should develop from just continuing to pass remarks like these between you and your spouse. Your kids should be used to this by now.

These gradual and planned approaches to the topic of masturbation should serve to reduce embarrassment and to reveal the interest of your kids that is likely already there.

Directing informal comments to your kids can be another way of opening intimate conversations about masturbation. Good conversation-starters to use here are the many masturbation myths that exist now or existed when you were growing up. For example, some kids have the misconception that masturbation causes acne or even blindness. Myths like these can easily be destroyed with a few lighthearted words. You might say, "When I was a kid people thought that masturbation would make you go blind. Can you believe that?" Or, you might comment, "Your skin seems to be clearing up lately. Did you know that some people think that masturbation causes acne? Pretty crazy, huh?" While correcting their possible misconceptions, your words and attitude will indicate your acceptance of talking about masturbation and even your acceptance of masturbation itself.

These seemingly innocent remarks from you about masturbation may stir your kids into opening up to you with questions and concerns. The outcome of this will be their awareness that masturbation *is* acceptable, that masturbation is not a "dirty" act, and that masturbation can offer a high degree of pleasure and be a very satisfactory, AIDS-safe alternative to interpersonal sex.

EPILOGUE ON ALTERNATIVES: NOTHING IS FOREVER

The decision to adopt alternatives to interpersonal sex won't be a static, unchanging one. Evolving circumstances, including evidence that your kids are no longer abstaining, will force you to consider teaching safer sex, as discussed in Part II of this book. Sooner or later your kids will likely need some good coaching in the use of condoms and some frank discussions and guidance on sexual alternatives to intercourse. Your successful promotion of alternatives to interpersonal sex, particularly masturbation, could provide you with a more open parental relationship, which is something that will be much-needed and appreciated as your children grow up. Your kids may also be more likely to keep you informed of their changing social/sexual situations and needs if you have open communication. Being able to talk with each other about previously sensitive and embarrassing topics can turn out to be one of the most constructive aspects of your family's relationship. It will certainly be one of the most important safeguards your kids can have from the risk of AIDS.

PART IV

Medical Considerations

9

AIDS: The Medical Facts

In order to discuss AIDS (Acquired Immune Deficiency Syndrome) with your kids it is necessary to understand several important aspects of the disease and the virus that causes it, as well as how AIDS is transmitted and what the likelihood is of contracting it through various behaviors. This information can help you to avoid high-risk behavior. Although the information discussed here is up-to-date as of the end of 1991, it is of paramount importance to be alert for new developments and findings that might require revision of behaviors designed to minimize risks.

THE DISEASE

While the AIDS problem tests the limits of scientists' knowledge of viruses, the scientific community has been loud and clear on one important issue: At this point we see no cure on the immediate horizon, and a safe, effective vaccine will likely remain a dream for the time being. We are told by the best scientific minds that education aimed at prevention is the best solution to AIDS-proof your children. Our society's ability to make mass behavior changes may well determine the future of our civilization.

127

Sadly, we can already see that the simple knowledge of facts and figures does not result in the required behavior changes. Therefore, the information in this chapter must not be viewed as sufficient in itself to protect your kids. Only if this information assists in bringing about protective behavior does it have any use at all. This chapter, however, can serve as a good starting place for the more intense education described in the other chapters and provides the facts for the required changes of behavior.

In AIDS-proofing your kids it is not important to learn all the detailed scientific information available on AIDS. It is more important that you make the decision to change behavior to protect your family from AIDS. The most important information is not difficult to learn and is found in the following discussion of AIDS. This chapter will explain:

- The way we relate to our biological world and how that is affected by AIDS

- The AIDS disease and when the virus is most easily transmitted

- The history of the AIDS epidemic in Africa and America and why it is significant

- Modes of transmission

- How to protect from the disease

- Treatments and vaccines.

Our Biological Environment

We share our biological world with numerous other types of living things, many of which find our bodies to be an ideal environment to inhabit. Some bacteria, for example, live in the intestinal tract in a cooperative manner with shared advantages. Many bacteria, fungi, and viruses, however, can live in or on us in a more aggressive manner, unnoticed until they find an opening. Once these organisms invade the body they can cause a great deal of harm.

The common yeast called *Candida albicans* is a good example. It is found frequently on the skin, but only occasionally causes problems such as diaper rash or thrush in babies and vaginal infections in women. Normally we don't suffer continuously from yeast infections, because our immune system becomes programmed to recognize and fight yeast, thus making the body an inhospitable place for it to grow. A similar situation prevails with many other organisms, and the battle between us and them goes on day and night for our entire lives.

The Immune System and AIDS

Ordinarily the immune system protects us from these common, potentially harmful invaders. This system is able to detect an invader and direct and carry out an attack against that invader. Immune-system cells mark and destroy foreign organisms when directed to do so by T4 helper cells. This battle, which goes on constantly without our being aware of it, prevents potential invaders from gaining the advantage over us.

Central to these immune-protection activities is a group of cells called T4 helper cells. These cells direct other cells to perform their specific functions as described above. Without T4 helper cells, our immune system would not be able to carry out the identification and neutralization activities described. In a person who is afflicted with AIDS, the T4 cells have been destroyed or functionally impaired by a very clever invader called the Human Immunodeficiency Virus (HIV). Acquired Immune Deficiency Syndrome (AIDS) is the result of immune impairment due to infection by HIV, which results in the destruction of the T4 helper cells. Without T4 helper cells, the other immune cells that normally produce antibodies or attack invaders directly never get the message to carry out their normal functions and the body can no longer defend itself against the many organisms struggling to take up residence within it. Infection by these organisms results in most of the symptoms of AIDS.

Carriers Can Infect Others Before They Have Symptoms

Long before any of the symptoms of AIDS are seen, a lot has already happened. The illness called AIDS represents only the terminal stage of prolonged infection by HIV. During most of the stages of HIV disease, the infected person generally has no symptoms and no outward signs of illness. The HIV carrier is often totally unaware that he or she has sustained a steady, persistent drop in the number of T4 helper cells over the course of several years. There are few symptoms and signs of disease until the number of T4 cells drops to a point at which their helper function no longer operates. At this point the immune system collapses, invaders start to take over, and AIDS symptoms appear. The difficult truth is that for a period ranging from months to years a person can be infected with HIV and thus able to pass it to someone else, but not be aware that they are spreading a fatal disease. We can not identify a carrier by appearance!

In the Beginning — No Symptoms, No Test

But, you ask, won't a test show if a person is infected or not? The answer to that is a definite maybe! At this time the two tests being given look for antibodies to HIV. These anti-bodies do not appear immediately on exposure to HIV, and thus a test is not a sure thing. This period when a carrier does not show a positive HIV antibody test usually varies from about six weeks to six months and rarely longer. This time period is called the "window phase." It is not possible to tell that a person is ill during this period. Some exposed persons, however, do recognize early nonspecific symptoms of viral infection.

Early Nonspecific Symptoms

We now know that some newly infected persons recognize typical viral symptoms on first exposure to HIV. These symptoms might include:
- Headache
- Fever
- Fatigue
- Swollen glands
- Rash.

There is nothing peculiar here to distinguish HIV from any of the dozens of other viruses, such as mononucleosis, which can cause similar symptoms. In a patient with early HIV disease, these symptoms usually last several weeks and then disappear, just as if any other virus were responsible. These signs are thus not reliable to serve as an early warning of HIV infection.

The Appearance of Symptoms

As the T4 helper cell level continues to decline over a period of months to years, the point is finally reached at which the director of the immune system can no longer perform its tasks and the immune system starts to collapse. There is the appearance of symptoms sometimes referred to as symptomatic HIV disease (previously known as ARC, or **AIDS R**elated Complex). These symptoms include such things as thrush (oral candida) or persistent herpes sores in the mouth or anus, but not the more serious systemic illnesses seen in AIDS. After another year or two, serious systemic diseases often develop in the infected person, and this is the point at which the condition is called AIDS.

AIDS, the Final Stage

The generalized systemic infections likely to be seen in this late stage are the result of the total disabling and destruction of the T4 cells. The immune system is now unable to protect at all from all those common organisms attempting to take up residence in the body. As we said before, we may not be aware of the constant immune battle going on within us, but if it suddenly stops, we certainly are going to know. Infections by organisms previously regarded as rare now become common, and the particular symptoms depend on which organisms are gaining the upper hand. For example:

- Weight loss often becomes extreme.
- Diarrhea is frequently intolerable.
- The skin is often severely attacked by infection or unusual cancers such as Kaposi's sarcoma.
- Profound fatigue may prevent the performance of normal work.
- A rare and severe form of pneumonia (PCP, or Pneumocystis Pneumonia) might appear.
- Death from severe infection can occur at any time.

AIDS is the Last Stage of HIV Disease

From the description you have just read concerning the usual course of infection due to HIV, you can now see that the term AIDS is far too limiting, in that AIDS represents only the terminal phase of a longer illness due to the virus called HIV. As you read the description of the HIV disease, we're certain some questions came to your mind. For example, the point at which an infected person is contagious is important to know, as is information on the duration of the initial "window phase" prior to a test becoming positive.

When Does an Infected Person Become Contagious?

Notice once again how long the time is from initial infection to the point at which the HIV antibody test becomes positive. The time needed to develop a positive test varies from about six weeks to six months after exposure to HIV, but in extremely rare cases it has taken as long as three years. This implies, of course, that all during that time a recently infected person could pass on the disease to others even though his or her antibody test is negative. This "window phase" is thought to be one of the periods of greatest risk for transmission, as there are too few antibodies to hold back the free viruses.

Then there is a longer period in which the infected person feels perfectly well and may not have any noticeable sign of the disease. This can go on for five, six, or seven years, and sometimes even longer! During this phase, scientists believe that few viruses are present and thus the patient is somewhat less infectious.

Following this prolonged interval, a second period of increased contagiousness is reached. These late stages see a dramatic drop in circulating antibodies as the immune system collapses with the disappearance of the T4 helper cells. This condition allows the accumulation of viruses and thus causes the patient to be more contagious once again. This second period of increased infectiousness includes the stage called AIDS.

What is important to remember is that no matter what phase the disease is in *a person infected with HIV is always contagious!* Precautions must always be taken.

Will All People with HIV Die of AIDS?

In the early days of the AIDS epidemic it was easy to misinterpret the AIDS mortality data. We were looking at the number of cases reported versus the number of deaths that had occurred up to that time. As the number of newly reported cases swelled dramatically, the illusion was that only some people would actually die of the disease. Studies done at the Walter Reed Institute followed a large number of patients and discovered that nearly all patients progressed from one stage to the next with time. Their conclusion is that the vast majority of persons infected with HIV will ultimately die from their condition, unless some useful therapy or a cure is found.

THE HISTORY OF AIDS

The North American Experience

Scientists now believe AIDS was introduced into North America in the mid- to late-1970s. The first twelve cases were described in 1981, and since then the number of cases has increased at an alarming rate. Initially, the outbreak was thought to be confined to homosexual males, but rapidly, as the means of transmission became understood, other groups came to be seen as having special risk. Recipients of blood and blood products were the second group found to be at risk, especially hemophiliacs. Third, the disease appeared in those people using intravenous (IV) drugs and sharing needles and syringes. Finally it appeared in people who had sexual contact with the first three groups. As more women became infected by these routes, it also appeared in babies born to infected mothers.

In spite of this movement of the disease into the heterosexual population, the North American public continues to hold the mistaken attitude that AIDS is primarily a homosexual disease. As we indicate below, however, the manner in which the disease is transmitted plainly shows that this disease can affect any group of sexually active people without regard to sexual orientation or gender. Further, a look at the African situation suggests that our North American style of defining narrow risk groups is a dangerous preoccupation, as we tend to avoid looking at our own risk behaviors while considering that AIDS is someone else's problem.

The African Situation

In Africa, AIDS has been around for a longer period of time. Scientists have found evidence of HIV in blood samples drawn as early as 1959. Thus Africa is at a more mature stage of the epidemic. By looking at their statistics we get an idea of what could happen here if adequate steps are not taken to control the spread of the disease. The most striking difference we see is that in Africa the sex ratio of infected males vs. females is at least equal, and in many places more women are infected than men. In Africa the most common means of contracting HIV is by heterosexual vaginal intercourse.

Already we see a shift in North America toward an increasing number of heterosexual cases of AIDS. It is very clear that unless we are able to make significant behavior changes now, we will ultimately face the horrendous problem seen in Africa, where so many people carry HIV that any sexual partner is a high-risk partner.

The Big Risk Group

With heterosexual vaginal intercourse being an important means of transmission worldwide, it follows that each person's risk of meeting an HIV carrier goes up with each sexual encounter. Those more at risk are sexually active young people who are not yet in lifelong monogamous relationships. This group represents tomorrow's general population. Should they become HIV-infected, we will experience Africa's dilemma.

How do we know this group is at special risk? Easy! We simply observe the prevalence of chlamydia, another disease that is passed on sexually in much the same way as HIV. Chlamydia, which often causes pelvic pain in women and mild penile discharge in men, is a good indicator of high-risk behavior because it has a short incubation period compared to AIDS. In other words, you don't need to wait years to see if you caught it or not. Currently, chlamydia is the most common sexually transmitted disease (STD) contracted by young people and is growing in epidemic proportions. If you use the growth of this STD to estimate the high-risk behavior that is taking place in this group, one must conclude that prevention techniques, techniques that would help protect kids from AIDS, are not being used reliably. As more people begin using these prevention techniques reliably, we will be able to measure our progress at reducing risk behavior in our communities by watching for a decrease in reports of chlamydia.

Preventing the invasion of AIDS into our young people at risk will prevent us from repeating Africa's experience. In order to do this it is the responsibility of each of us to see that every person close to us has the information and training necessary to minimize his or her risk. High-risk behaviors can be better understood and avoided if we clearly understand how HIV is transmitted.

HOW THE AIDS VIRUS IS TRANSMITTED

HIV, the AIDS virus, is fortunately not a very tough virus when out of the body. This means that very close contact must be made in order for it to be passed from one person to the next. It cannot be passed from floating in the air like the measles virus or by coughing in a person's face. Because it is normally found in certain blood cells, the easiest way to pass it is to transfer blood from person to person, as happens when having a blood transfusion. Fortunately, through careful testing of donor blood and by behavioral screening of blood donors themselves, the risk of becoming infected in this way is now very small. Nevertheless, those individuals who received blood before 1985 should ask their doctor if an HIV antibody test should be done.

Few of us will actually ever need to have a blood transfusion, but blood is also passed from person to person by IV drug users sharing needles and syringes. People engaged in this high-risk activity should be regarded as carriers of HIV regardless of their antibody test results because the test is not dependable due to their more recent exposures.

Other bodily fluids are also able to carry the virus. Semen and vaginal secretions have proven to be effective fluids in which to pass HIV. Furthermore, cells lining the vagina and rectum have receptor sites for the virus. These are attachment sites on the surface of cells that bind with the virus, increasing its chance of entering the body. This explains why both vaginal intercourse for women and receptive anal intercourse for either sex are such efficient ways of spreading HIV and why special precautions have to be taken to protect our families from these dangerous types of sexual activities.

It is less likely for a male to become infected with HIV via vaginal intercourse with an infected woman or via anal intercourse with an infected partner of either sex. Various studies suggest there is a twofold to fourfold increase in risk for the receptive partner. Over the span of one's sexual life this difference is not likely to be significant, because it is really only a matter of timing — it can happen sooner or later.

Other means of passing the AIDS virus are also possible though less probable. Recently, for example, there have been athletes who, in order to cheat on urine tests for drug screening, used a catheter to insert someone else's urine into their own bladder. Urine frequently has both white and red blood cells in it, so this is a dangerous activity. This case illustrates the need for people to think about their own activities, assess their individual risks, and modify their behavior as needed.

For most of us the most dangerous behaviors involve sexual contact with a carrier. To be overly concerned with theoretical but extremely rare modes of HIV transmission is a lot like standing blindfolded in the middle of a freeway while expressing concern about being struck by lightning. We will, therefore, not be concerned that biting, scratching, or insect bites are a risk. They are not! For the vast majority of us, excluding IV drug users and blood-product users, the real danger is from unprotected vaginal or anal intercourse and oral sex with someone infected by HIV.

The Spread of HIV by Sexual Contact

Sexual contact is the most likely means of contracting the AIDS virus, as well as the easiest way to pass it on to someone else. There is no doubt that sexual intercourse — either heterosexual or homosexual — can pass the virus from person to person very easily. All that is required is intimate contact without condoms with one infected partner. Remember that carriers look perfectly healthy and usually are unaware that they are carrying this deadly virus.

Are there any sexual practices that are more dangerous than others? Yes, we can say that some sexual interactions are more likely to pass the virus than others. For example, anal intercourse is slightly more risky, if one person is a carrier, than is vaginal intercourse. The difference, however, is not great.

Anal intercourse is the most risky homosexual behavior, but if you think that it is a behavior confined to homosexuals, let us point out that heterosexual persons in every generation discover for themselves that pregnancy doesn't happen this way, and thus, at some time or another, many heterosexuals practice this as a form of birth control, as well as a pleasurable sexual option. Remember, however, that anal intercourse does hold the distinction of being the most likely means of passing the AIDS virus of any sexual behavior. Homosexual men who practice safer sex usually feel more secure using two condoms for this activity. Heterosexuals should be just as careful or avoid it altogether.

Vaginal or anal sex with proper and practiced condom use is considered activity of intermediate-risk. The precise risk has to take into consideration the skill of the condom user as well as the screening of the prospective partner. The skills taught in Chapter 4 of this book are designed to minimize the risk of these otherwise risky activities, which sooner or later nearly all people take part in.

Some forms of sexual activity are classified as low-risk because transmission of HIV, while possible, is not likely in these ways. Oral sex, for example, is often used as an alternative to vaginal intercourse, not only because it can be a pleasurable experience, but also for reasons of birth control. What can we say about HIV transfer during oral sex? We do know of a few cases where HIV has apparently been passed on during oral sex. As mentioned in Chapter 5, the precise

The Spectrum of Risk

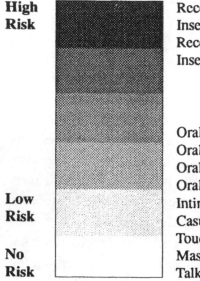

High Risk — Receptive anal intercourse
Insertive anal intercourse
Receptive vaginal intercourse
Insertive vaginal intercourse

Oral sex on a man with ejaculation
Oral sex on a man without ejaculation
Oral sex on a woman
Oral-anal contact

Low Risk — Intimate kissing
Casual kissing
Touching, massage

No Risk — Masturbation
Talking, fantasy

Courtesy of the American College Health Association

risk of oral sex varies with the particular situation. The presence of vaginal or oral bleeding increases the risk of HIV transmission. You wouldn't want to be the unlucky person who contracts the AIDS virus this way. You will get just as sick if you get AIDS a less common way as if you get it through a very dangerous activity. Therefore, condoms or other suitable protective devices should always be used for this activity as well as for vaginal and anal intercourse. Contact your local AIDS organization for advice.

Deep or wet kissing is also considered a low-risk activity, but keep in mind that other factors which cause the exchange of blood will increase the risk. For example, the presence of a herpes cold sore in one person and a recent tooth extraction in the other could allow the passage of HIV. In other words, it's important to use common sense applied to the knowledge of how transmission happens.

Now the good news: Safe forms of human contact are possible for those who choose abstinence and for all people during the early stages of forming a relationship and learning about the partner's past. Hugging, petting, massage, and dry kissing are safe. You cannot acquire HIV from a carrier by these activities.

HOW TO PROTECT FROM AIDS

How Many HIV Carriers Are in Your Community?

An excellent topic for your kids to study concerns the impact of AIDS in your community. Information can be obtained from your local public health office on the number of AIDS cases in your area. This year's information on how many have been infected can be compared to last year's and then projections can be made for next year. This could be an instructive topic for a school report.

Your kids will become interested in the many problems associated with AIDS, such as discrimination and escalating healthcare costs, and most importantly will feel they made some discoveries on their own. Knowledge acquired in this manner is generally more likely to lead to required lifestyle changes than information received in a passive manner. Keeping in touch with the changing statistics will keep you abreast of the success your community is having in AIDS-prevention programs.

As mentioned earlier, following the number of new cases of chlamydia or other STDs is also a good way of assessing the success of your prevention programs. Some of your friends, for example, might not see the need for the kind of explicit instruction advocated in this book. If young people in your community are being diagnosed with chlamydia or other STDs, however, this is evidence enough that the door is open for HIV. Ask your public health office about the incidence of various STDs in your community.

Partner Selection and Screening — Before the Condom

In order to minimize risk of exposure to HIV it is important to consider first the risk of your potential partner. This should be done before any contact that might allow passage of the AIDS virus. This means that you must know whether IV drugs were used in the past and how many partners that person has been with in the past and what their risks were. Even geographic location is important, as some communities with greater numbers of carriers have correspondingly greater risks. You need to know how your partners have interacted with any high-risk groups or if they have engaged in any high-risk behaviors.

Finally, you must realize that even after you are as sure as humanly possible about the safety of your partner, you can never be absolutely certain. This fact is borne out in STD clinics everywhere, where the lesson is learned over and over again that the truth about your partner's past is so often known only after a disease has been transmitted. Many people today opt for an HIV antibody test to prove to their partner and to themselves that they are safe. This is of help too, but you must remember to abstain from all risky behavior for a period of six months prior to taking the test, because testing in that silent "window phase" of HIV infection does not give an accurate picture of possible infection. The use of condoms can add an extra margin of safety that could be life-saving, but only after you have also carefully screened your partner.

The Importance of Condom Use

Scientific evidence continues to support the notion that condoms, used consistently and properly, are useful in preventing the spread of HIV as well as other sexually transmitted diseases. It is important to realize that no matter how careful and well-prepared we are, nothing is infallible. Thus we emphasize the point that condoms will only make *a safe partner safer and a dangerous partner less dangerous.*

The Importance of a Clear Head

Finally, because great thought and care are required to ensure safety during sexual activity, from partner selection and limiting our lifetime number of partners to the mechanics of condom use itself, it should be apparent that this is no time for a cloudy mind. Just as we have taught our kids the importance of not driving when drinking, we should teach them the same thing about sexual intercourse. *If you've been drinking or taking other drugs, do not have sex—make no exceptions.* It has been our professional experience that substance abuse *frequently* precedes unplanned intercourse followed by unintended pregnancy and STDs.

Summary of Steps to Avoid AIDS

- Understand how HIV is transmitted.

- Keep up-to-date with new findings that might alter your risks.

- Practice talking to your partners about their pasts, and practice talking about and assessing high-risk behavior.

- Get as much mileage as possible from the safer sex activities described. Limit your partners to as small a number as possible.

- Before engaging in sexual intercourse, learn the art of using condoms effectively. Learn the methods of handling condoms before, during and after use.

- Understand the relationship between drug and alcohol use and high-risk behavior. Resolve never to engage in sexual activity while under the influence of alcohol or other drugs.

TREATMENTS AND VACCINES

Is There Hope for the Future?

Remember the days not long ago when war was declared on cancer? The idea seemed to be that if we dump enough money on enough scientists any problem can be solved! But nothing is a sure thing, and we are now witnessing a repetition of that war on cancer in the new war on AIDS. The results will likely be the same: new hopes every few months that the newest experimental drug will prove to be the elusive magic bullet.

The most we can reasonably hope for on the chemical warfare front is more of what we have already seen. New drugs will surely postpone death and even make life more bearable and productive for persons with HIV disease. The possibility of a total cure, however, is too far in the future to rely on it for AIDS-proofing your kids. While news of possible treatments and cures may sound promising to you, remember that they do nothing to slow the spread of HIV.

While the national preoccupation with a search for the cure consumes the lion's share of our money for AIDS, effort spent on effective preventive programs for this disease go begging. Considering that this disease, due to its limited means of spread, is now totally preventable, we must ask why the emphasis hasn't been put on prevention?

Will There Be a Vaccine?

Can the epidemic be stopped by a vaccine designed to boost one's immunity to HIV before making contact? Theoretically yes, but don't hold your breath waiting. Optimists point to the astonishing success achieved in eradicating smallpox by vaccination. Smallpox, however, is the only complete success story to date. In the case of smallpox, nature already provided for us the protective virus in the form of the cowpox virus. With HIV no such protective virus has been found.

On the positive side, scientists today can manipulate viruses and the immune system in new ways, and the possibility does exist that some engineered vaccine will prove usable in the future. Such developments, while proceeding, are still over the horizon.

You Are On Your Own

In this situation we must be fully aware that the ability of governments to help is rather limited. The best they can do today is give us information. The avoidance of HIV and AIDS is totally up to each individual, and that will likely be the situation for the foreseeable future. This makes the information in this book all the more important.

PART V

Extra Benefits, Further Readings and Groups to Contact

10

Extra Benefits from AIDS-Proofing

The problems of AIDS-proofing your kids are really not very different from the general problems of parenting. This is especially true for such potentially sensitive issues as dating and socializing; schooling; alcohol, drug, and tobacco use; personal and family responsibilities; and a myriad of other issues that may be relevant in your home. Progressive coaching, realistic practice, and the generous provision of praise and rewards will be helpful in all areas of parenting.

Anything that your kids are not doing which you think is important for them to do can benefit from these parenting tools. Whether you feel that your kids are not doing something desirable because they're too lazy, too afraid or anxious, lacking in skills, or just not interested, you can take effective, positive action. You can help build behavior.

In learning how to effectively AIDS-proof your kids, you've learned that:

- You should proceed slowly when teaching them new, difficult habits.

- Parental instruction should begin at a level your kids can succeed at and progress from there.

- This progression must be rich in praise, encouragement, and even material rewards when needed.

- Habits must be practiced, and practiced under as realistic conditions as possible, if they're to be counted on to occur when needed.

YOU'LL BE A MORE POSITIVE, LIKABLE PARENT

Most importantly, there's been an extra benefit to using the parenting techniques we've advocated. If you've already begun AIDS-proofing, then perhaps you've noticed that there's been little need for threats, nagging, or other negative and coercive reactions. Progressive coaching had you start at your kids' current level of competence and build from there rather than nag or plead for skills they weren't as yet showing. You haven't had to demand, outright, what they should be doing. Instead, you've been working toward what they *should be* doing by building on what they *are* doing. This has maximized your kids' successes, allowing you to be a welcomed and valued source of positive reactions.

As a result of your positive reactions, instead of nagging, scolding, and threats, you've likely become an increasingly trusted and reliable resource for your kids. And you've undoubtedly become a more likable parent.

YOU'LL BE A MORE EFFECTIVE PARENT

You can continue to be a valuable resource to your kids by extending what you've learned in AIDS-proofing your kids to other sensitive issues in parenting.

Alcohol Use

You can help to teach your kids to use alcohol in safe ways or to abstain from alcohol use altogether. The issues and techniques are the same as for the delicate problem of AIDS.

Safe drinking means more than just knowing when and where to do it. It means learning specific skills.

- Do it responsibly, under safe and acceptable conditions.

- Drink only moderate amounts and refuse any more in spite of urgings from friends.

- Call a taxi or catch a bus home.

- Practice these skills under realistic conditions with adequate encouragement and incentives.

Abstinence may be your goal if your values or situation requires that your kids defer drinking during this period of their lives. If abstinence is the goal, then abstinence from alcohol means your kids must have the skill to assert their refusal of alcoholic drinks in social situations under conditions of increasing peer pressure. It also means promoting your kids' involvement with social groups and activities where drinking isn't done. You know the function of progressive coaching, realistic practice, role-plays, and the generous use of praise and rewards. The details bear a remarkable similarity to AIDS-proofing.

Drug Use

We hope that your kids never get into drugs. We have no idea, however, of your drug habits, nor do we know to what extent the social use of drugs is condoned in your family or circle of friends. We do know that the so-called "soft" drugs are more widely used by adults in our culture than most would like to admit. The issues and problems for controlling your kids' use of drugs are the same as for drinking and sexual practices.

If you want your kids to abstain from drug use, you'll have to teach them the skills that will permit this.

- Be active in helping them find "safe" social activities and social groups.

- Give them the assertive verbal skills to effectively refuse drug experimentation with other kids.

- Practice with realistic role-plays to develop your kids' assertiveness.

- Rehearse, rehearse, rehearse, so that these responses will come naturally and in a style appropriate to their peer group.

We hope abstinence will be your choice. If some drug use is to be tolerated or accepted by you, then you'll have to consider teaching your kids how to use drugs with a minimum of health risk. The role of heavy doses or extended use in the incidence of strokes, lung disease, road and pedestrian accidents, carelessness in sex practices, and other outcomes must be considered.

In the case of "hard" drugs, the transmission of AIDS by the use of shared needles is well-documented. You will, of course, be anxious if your kids associate with anyone using "hard" drugs, not only because you want your kids to avoid forming such a treacherous habit, but because sexual encounters with members of this high-risk group would increase the chance of your kids contracting AIDS.

The problem of drug use, of course, is a topic for another entire book, but you should see the relevance of the issues and techniques covered in this book.

OTHER PARENTING PROBLEMS

Many of your concerns as a parent have to do with developing responsible behaviors in your kids, behaviors that demonstrate consideration of others and consideration of your kids' own long-term interests.

Here are some examples of unending parental quests that should strike a familiar chord with you:

- Regularly saving part of their earnings or allowance

- Being polite and sociable with family, family friends, and other adults

- Helping around the house with a smile

You may consider this to be "pie-in-the-sky" wishful thinking. You may have attempted to instill these good habits by using thinly veiled threats, nagging, pleading, or outright demands. These could work, but there are better ways.

In all these cases, the answer is the same as before. Move comfortably into the required behavior. Some kids — more likely the younger ones — may be quite intimidated by new adult-type responsibilities. A bank, for example, with line-ups of busy adults, forms to fill out, vault doors, and armed guards, may provide more than a few anxious moments. You can help your kids by giving them some preparation under more relaxed, less public conditions at home. (Role-play how one opens a savings account. Bring some deposit slips home from the bank so that your kids can learn how to fill them out.)

Build their savings skills gradually. Begin with a level of regular savings they can easily live with (_____ dollars a month), raise standards slowly (increasing to _____ dollars over the next several months), and be supportive and rewarding (accompany their deposits with your own percentage contribution to the total).

For many responsible, adult-like behaviors, including the sexually oriented behaviors this book has been concerned with, it is helpful if you begin coaching behaviors as early as possible. The more opportunity your kids have to develop undesirable habits, the harder it will be to replace these habits with better ones. As a general rule, it is much easier to develop new habits than to get rid of old ones.

It's all a matter of selecting your goal, beginning with a comfortable, easily attained approximation to it, keeping spirits high with praise and rewards, and building success upon success. We've suggested further readings on this technology of behavior management at the end of this chapter.

AVOIDING THE THREAT-
AND-PUNISHMENT TRAP

As we said earlier, if you've followed the steps in this book faithfully, you've had no need for threatening, scolding, nagging, pleading, or laying down "guilt trips" or "grounding" your kids. Parenting that promotes close and warm family relationships is always preferred. The effective and generous use of praise and rewards, not threats and punishment, will do this.

In spite of one's best intentions, however, it's not hard to fall into the trap of relying on threats and punishment. It would be foolish to pretend otherwise and even more foolish to fail to understand the reasons for these mistakes — and they are mistakes. Not only do threatening, scolding, nagging, pleading, and other instructional attempts like these feel bad for everyone, they don't create long-lasting, desirable changes. All too soon, parents find themselves repeating the use of threats and punishment over and over again.

WHY ARE THREATS AND PUNISHMENT
SO TEMPTING TO USE?

Why do we, as parents, succumb to the use of threats and punishment? Surely parents — most of us, anyway — do not enjoy treating kids this way. Threats and punishment are used, unfortunately, because of their immediate effects.

There is no quicker way to bring about sudden and dramatic but temporary changes in kids' behavior than to swing a sufficiently frightening "stick," whether in word or deed. And though parents would wish for more permanent changes in behavior, it is their kids' compliance, for the moment, that is so rewarding to the parent swinging the stick. This is the trap! Because of these immediate effects, parents are unfortunately rewarded for using punishments or threats that, in the long run, are ineffective.

We don't wish to suggest that there aren't times when a quick, effective threat or punishment is called for. Kids can sometimes do things that are very harmful to themselves or others. Your child has, perhaps, just run across the street against a red light, not noticing the panicked motorist who swerved to miss her. At times like this, if you're there when it happens, the reaction from a concerned parent may justifiably be an immediately negative one. But don't forget the spirit of this book: *An ounce of prevention is worth a pound of cure*. As with the risks of AIDS, the way to handle this problem would be to effectively traffic-proof your kids.

REWARD VS. PUNISHMENT

The hollow promise of success will, as we've said, tempt you to use threats and punishment. And the illusion of success can trap you into even more frequent threats and punishment. Moreover, the use of progressive coaching and realistic practice with praise and reward throughout is costlier than punishment in time, effort, and family resources. The scales may seem to favor your use of threats and punishment, but it's an illusion. This is why we're taking the time to point out that building change with positive reactions is healthier. The results are more permanent and they feel a whole lot better for you, your kids, and the entire family.

To summarize, throughout this book we've attempted to teach you to use the "carrot" rather than the "stick." We've advocated that you:

- Initially only require behaviors from your kids that they can already do successfully, so that you can be a source of praise and reward right from the beginning.

- Increase your requirements on your kids in small steps so that you'll build upon success and continue to be a generous source of encouragement and reward.

- Use realistic practice and role-plays and be obvious and explicit in showing your appreciation, approval, and support for your kids' smallest accomplishments.

This is the road that effectively builds your kids' skills in sensitive areas while minimizing discomforts and embarrassments, which is especially important with the very difficult issue of AIDS-proofing. Your having traveled this road with your kids will make you better prepared for the many other sensitive family problems that can be solved by effective parenting.

Further Readings

A Kid's First Book about Sex. Joani Blank and Marcia Quackenbush. Burlingame, Calif.: Yes Press [Down There Press], 1983. Toronto, Ontario: Kids Can Press.

Cartoon illustrations and text. Directed at preteens and young teens, but suitable for all. A general sex-education book that clarifies experiences of feeling aroused, masturbating, and having an orgasm, and also covers popular terms for basic sexual activities.

Assets: Social Skills for Adolescents. Dr. J. S. Hazel et al. Champaign, Ill.: Research Press.

Video or film. Expensive but excellent. Designed for school use. Includes learning how to say "no," resisting peer pressure, resolving conflicts with others, expressing and accepting criticism, and other skills.

Becoming Orgasmic: A Sexual Growth Program for Women. Julia Heiman, Leslie LoPiccolo, and Joseph LoPiccolo. Englewood Cliffs, N.J.: Prentice-Hall, 1976.

Describes a number of ways for women to increase their sexual enjoyment either by themselves or with a partner.

Behavior Modification: What It Is and How to Do It.
Dr. Garry Martin and Dr. Joseph Pear. Englewood Cliffs,
N.J.: Prentice-Hall, 1988.
> *Thorough and readable. For parents and professionals,
> with emphasis on kids with problems.*

Consumer Reports. Consumers Union of the United
States. N.Y.
> *Available at magazine outlets. Consult back and future
> issues for ongoing reports on sexual hygiene products and
> medical updates on AIDS-related matters.*

Families: Application of Social Learning to Family Life.
Gerald R. Patterson. Waterloo, Ontario, Canada: Research
Press, 1975.
> *Basic behavioral parenting book. Easy to read and
> understand.*

For Yourself: The Fulfillment of Sexuality. Lonnie
Garfield Barbach. Garden City, N.Y.: Anchor Books
[Doubleday], 1976.
> *See description of* Becoming Orgasmic: A Sexual Growth
> Program for Women.

Principles of Everyday Behavior Analysis. Dr. L. Keith
Miller. Pacific Grove, Calif.: Brooks/Cole, 1980.
> *Thorough and readable. A basic book in behavior analy-
> sis for parents and professionals.*

Safer Sex Guidelines. Toronto, Ontario: Canadian AIDS
Society.
> *A detailed report on the relative risks for AIDS of various
> sexual practices and techniques.*

The Joy of Sex. Alex Comfort. New York: Fireside [Simon & Schuster], 1974.

Describes a wide variety of sexual activities that couples can share in a loving and enjoyable way, including many alternatives to intercourse.

The New Teenage Body Book. Kathy McCoy and Charles Wibblesman, M.D. Los Angeles: Body Press [Price Stern Sloan], 1987.

Directed at teenage readers, but equally important for parents. Includes advice in letters from teens on sensitive sexual issues such as masturbation, sexual preferences, intercourse, diseases, and contraception.

Where Did I Come From?: The Facts of Life without any Nonsense and with Illustrations. Peter Mayle. Secaucus, N.J.: Lyle Stuart [Carol Publishing Group], 1975.

Humorously illustrated. Directed at preteens, but suitable and entertaining for all. Includes an excellent introduction to intercourse.

Groups to Contact for More Information

TELEPHONE HOTLINES IN THE UNITED STATES

National AIDS Hotline

1-800-342-2437 (toll-free)

Supplies information about AIDS and gives referrals to local groups for further services.

Linea Nacional de SIDA

1-800-344-SIDA (toll-free)

For Spanish-speaking persons.

TTY/TTD Hotline

1-800-AIDS-TTY (toll-free)

For hearing-impaired persons.

National AIDS Information Clearing House

1-800-458-5231 (toll-free)

Supplies informative booklets, videos, and programs on AIDS for businesses and schools.

STD National Hotline

1-800-227-8922

Supplies information on all sexually transmitted diseases, including AIDS.

163

ORGANIZATIONS IN THE UNITED STATES

American College Health Association
P.O. Box 28937
Baltimore, MD 21240-8937
(410) 859-1500

Puts out many informative pamphlets on safer sex and AIDS.

American Social Health Association
P.O. Box 13827
Research Triangle Park, NC 27709
(919) 361-8425

Puts out many informative pamphlets on sexually trans-mitted diseases, including AIDS.

National AIDS Interfaith Network
300 "I" St., N.E.
Washington, D.C. 20002
(202) 546-0807

Coalition of AIDS ministries and religious organizations, provides religious/spiritual support to people with AIDS and those concerned about the disease.

National Center for Health Education
72 Spring Street, Suite 208
New York, NY 10012
(212) 334-9470

Provides comprehensive health education curriculum, Growing Healthy®, *including AIDS information, for grades K-6, and also offers parent guide on AIDS prevention.*

National Minority AIDS Council
300 "I" St., N.E.
Washington, D.C. 20002
(202) 544-1076
> *Organizes and develops AIDS leadership groups in mi-*
> *nority communities, and puts out pamphlets on AIDS and*
> *its effects on minorities.*

Pediatric AIDS Foundation
1311 Colorado Avenue
Santa Monica, CA 90404
(213) 395-9051
> *Focuses on children with AIDS.*

San Francisco AIDS Foundation
24 Van Ness Avenue, 6th floor
San Francisco, CA 94102
(415) 863-AIDS
> *Puts out many informative pamphlets and is one of the old-*
> *est and most established AIDS organizations in the United*
> *States.*

Sex Information and Education Council of the United States (SIECUS)
130 W. 42nd Street, Suite 2500
New York, NY 10036
(212) 819-9770
> *Puts out pamphlets on all aspects of human sexuality, in-*
> *cluding AIDS, and offers access to their extensive library*
> *and information services.*

The Wedge Program
1540 Market Street, Suite 435
San Francisco, CA 94102
(415) 554-9098
> *This progressive high school/middle school program teaches about AIDS and prevention and could be used as a possible model in your area.*

Other sources of help and information:
Your local chapter of the American Red Cross
Your local Planned Parenthood clinic
Your doctor, school nurse, or other healthcare worker
Your local or state public health department
Your local AIDS service organization

TELEPHONE HOTLINES IN CANADA

Alberta Health — STD Control
(403) 427-2830 (Edmonton)
1-800-772-AIDS (throughout Alberta)

British Columbia Ministry of Health
(604) 872-6652 (Vancouver)
1-800-972-2437 (throughout British Columbia)

Manitoba Department of Health AIDS Infoline
(204) 945-AIDS (Winnipeg)
1-800-782-AIDS (throughout Manitoba)

Newfoundland Department of Health Disease Control
(709) 576-3430

New Brunswick
Department of Health: (506) 453-2536
AIDS New Brunswick: (506) 459-7518
   1-800-561-4009 (throughout New Brunswick)

Northwest Territories AIDS Information Line
(403) 873-7017
1-800-661-0795 (throughout the Northwest Territories)

Nova Scotia Department of Health,
Epidemiology Division
(902) 424-8698

Ontario Ministry of Health, AIDS Section
(416) 668-6066
English & other languages:
   1-800-668-2437 (throughout Ontario)
French: 1-800-267-7432 (throughout Ontario)

Prince Edward Island Department of Health
(902) 368-4530

Quebec Department of Health
(418) 643-9395
1-800-463-5656 (throughout Quebec)

Saskatchewan Health Education Line
(306) 787-3148
1-800-667-7766 (throughout Saskatchewan)

Yukon Ministry of Health
(403) 668-9444 (Whitehorse)
1-800-661-0507 (throughout Yukon)

ORGANIZATIONS IN CANADA

Canadian Public Health Association:
AIDS Education and Awareness Program
400-1565 Carling Avenue
Ottawa, Ontario K1Z 8R1
(613) 725-3769
> *Puts out many informative pamphlets and videos on safer sex and AIDS.*

Federal Center for AIDS
301 Elgin Street
Ottawa, Ontario K1A 0L2
(613) 957-1772
> *Puts out many informative pamphlets and videos on safer sex and AIDS.*

Other sources of help and information:
Your Public Health Unit or Community Health Centre
Your local AIDS service organization
Your Provincial Ministry of Health
Your doctor

Other Books of Interest Available From Beyond Words Publishing, Inc.

DARE TO LIVE
Author: Michael Miller
257 pages, 5.5 x 8.5 inches, $9.95 softbound
An upbeat, practical look at recognizing, understanding and preventing teen depression and suicide; written for adults, parents, counselors and teens. Michael Miller is nationally recognized for his work with young people and his school programs in the area of suicide prevention.

TRIUMPH OVER DARKNESS
Author: Wendy Wood
294 pages, 8 x 9.5 inches, $12.95, softbound
A book geared toward understanding and healing the trauma of childhood sexual abuse. A collection of powerful commentaries of incest, rape, and abuse. Through poetry, art, powerful commentaries and personal accounts, 70 women share their varied experiences of childhood sexual abuse and their healing process.

RAISING A SON: Parents and the Making of a Healthy Man
Authors: Don and Jeanne Elium
225 pages, 6 .5 X 9 .5, $18.95 hardbound, $10.95 softbound
This conversationally-styled, "how-to" book, written by family counselors, is a guide to assist both mother and father in the parts they must play in the making of a healthy, assertive, and loving man. It is readable for parents, professional care providers and educators.

BETTER THAN A LEMONADE STAND:
50 Small Business Ideas for Kids
Author: Daryl Bernstein, $7.95 softbound, June 1992
Written by a 15-year old who has started and run his own small businesses since the age of eight. A self-proclaimed expert in this field, the author outlines directions for kids on how to start a small business, attract customers, maintain good customer relations, and expand the business. He writes in an easy-to-understand language for kids ages 8-16.

To order or to receive a catalog contact:
Beyond Words Publishing, Inc.
13950 NW Pumpkin Ridge Rd.
Hillsboro, OR 97123
(503) 647-5109 or toll-free: 1-800-284-9673